YOGA WITH A PARTNER

YOGA WITH A PARTNER

SANDRA JORDAN

Photographs: Sandra Jordan with Don Hallock

ARCO PUBLISHING, INC.
219 PARK AVENUE SOUTH, NEW YORK, N.Y. 10003

Published by Arco Publishing, Inc.
219 Park Avenue South, New York, New York 10003

Library of Congress Cataloging in Publication Data

Jordan, Sandra.
  Yoga with a partner.

  Bibliography: p.
  1. Yoga, Hatha. I. Title.
RA781.7.J65   613.7   79-24425

ISBN 0-668-04871-9 (Paper Edition)

Printed in the United States of America

For my friends,
  who help me see
  into my self.

CONTENTS

LIST OF ILLUSTRATIONS   8

PREFACE   11

INTRODUCTION   13

HOW TO BEGIN   15

THE PARTNERS   16
    Aeja Lee and Glenn Kawana

CHAPTER ONE: SITTING POSTURES   19
    Butterfly I (Baddha Konasana I)   20
    Butterfly I (Baddha Konasana I)
      Variation   22
    Butterfly II (Baddha Konasana II) 24
    Butterfly III (Baddha Konasana III) 26
    Butterfly II (Baddha Konasana II)
      Variation   28

CHAPTER TWO: FORWARD BENDING POSTURES   31
    Double Downward Dog Posture
      (Adho Mukha Svanasana) 32
    Bent Leg Forward Bend Pose I
      (Janu Sirsasana I)   34
    Bent Leg Forward Bend Pose II
      (Janu Sirsasana II)   36
    Straight Leg Forward Bend Pose I
      (Paschimottanasana I) 38
    Straight Leg Forward Bend Pose II
      (Paschimottanasana II) 40
    Straight Leg Forward Bend Pose III
      (Paschimottanasana III) 42
    Standing Forward Bend Pose (Uttanasana) 44

CHAPTER THREE: SIDE STRETCHES OF THE BODY
           AND INNER LEGS   47

    Beam Posture (Parighasana)   48

    Standing Leg Stretch (Utthita Padangustasana)   50

    Wide Angle Leg Stretch (Konasana)   52

CHAPTER FOUR: BACKBENDING POSTURES   54

    Chest Expansion Posture
      (Prasarita Padottanasana)   56

    Camel Posture I (Ustrasana I)   58

    Camel Posture II (Ustrasana II)   60

    Extended Cobra Pose (Bhujangasana)   62

    Bow Posture (Dhanurasana)   64

    Wheel Posture I (Urdhva Dhanurasana I)   66

    Wheel Posture II (Urdhva Dhanurasana II)   68

CHAPTER FIVE: INVERTED POSTURES   71

    Shoulderstand (Salamba Sarvangasana)   72

    Plough Posture (Halasana)   74

CHAPTER SIX: INTEGRATION AND INVENTION IN YOGA   77

    Breathing Awareness   79

      Basic Deep Breathing – The Complete Breath   81

    Developing Mindfullness Through Breath Awareness   83

      Breath Awareness Practice   85

    Deep Relaxation   87

      Deep Relaxation Pose (Savasana)   88

    Integration   91

    Experimentation   92

    Growth   93

SPECIAL REFERENCES   94

ILLUSTRATIONS

Full Lotus Posture (Padmasana). Advanced Pose.   16
Warrior's Posture (Virasana). Beginning Pose.   17
Butterfly I (Baddha Konasana I). Beginning Pose.   20
Butterfly I (Baddha Konasana I) Variation. Beginning Pose.   22
Butterfly II (Baddha Konasana II). Intermediate Pose.   24
Butterfly III (Baddha Konasana III). Advanced Pose.   26
Butterfly II (Baddha Konasana II) Variation. Intermediate Pose.   28
Double Downward Dog Posture (Adho Mukha Svanasana). Beginning Pose.   32
Bent Leg Forward Bend Pose I (Janu Sirsasana I). Beginning Pose.   34
Bent Leg Forward Bend Pose II (Janu Sirsasana II). Intermediate Pose.   36
Straight Leg Forward Bend Pose I (Paschimottanasana I). Beginning Pose.   38
Straight Leg Forward Bend Pose II (Paschimottanasana II). Beginning Pose.   40
Straight Leg Forward Bend Pose III (Paschimottanasana III). Intermediate Pose.   42
Standing Forward Bend Pose (Uttanasana). Advanced Pose.   44
Beam Posture (Parighasana). Beginning Pose.   48
Standing Leg Stretch (Utthita Padangusthasana). Intermediate Pose.   50
Wide Angle Leg Stretch (Konasana). Beginning Pose.   52
Chest Expansion Posture (Prasarita Padottanasana). Beginning Pose.   56
Camel Posture I (Ustrasana I). Beginning Pose.   58
Camel Posture II (Ustrasana II). Intermediate Pose.   60
Extended Cobra Pose (Bhujangasana). Beginning Pose.   62
Bow Posture (Dhanurasana). Intermediate Pose.   64
Wheel Posture I (Urdhva Dhanurasana I). Intermediate Pose.   66
Wheel Posture II (Urdhva Dhanurasana II). Advanced Pose.   68
Shoulderstand (Salamba Sarvangasana). Beginning Pose.   72
Plough Posture (Halasana). Intermediate Pose.   74

"One of the highest blessings
is a friend with whom
we can respond
openly and freely."

A. Sujata, BEGINNING TO SEE

PREFACE

I would like to gratefully acknowledge the students of Mr. B.K.S. Iyengar of India for their influence on my personal practice and teaching of Hatha Yoga. From my teachers I have learned the need to develop a solid foundation in the basic principles of Yoga before any postures can be clearly and safely communicated to others. It is my hope to one day have the opportunity to study with Mr. Iyengar in India.

This book is not intended to be a treatise on Yoga. Instead, it is meant to be a personal, creative experiment in developing our potential for growth through working with a friend.

INTRODUCTION

This book grew out of the creative, and often humorous, attempts of Yoga students to help their friends with their Yoga postures. Traditionally, Yoga is practiced alone or in a classroom led by a teacher. This book attempts to explore, illustrate and explain a new way of enjoying Yoga. By creating Yoga postures together, the friends in this book gained new insights, deepened their friendship, and thoroughly enjoyed themselves. Partnering removed the distinction between teacher and student, freed the friends to be creative, to experiment with new variations, and to become aware of the seemingly endless ways of working one body against another.

The goal of doing Yoga with a friend is to teach us more about ourselves, our own inner creativity, our capacity for fun, and our ability to relate in a free and natural way to one another.

HOW TO BEGIN

First of all choose a friend, male or female, you enjoy. The friendship is more important than flexibility or knowledge of Yoga. Ask a friend who wants to give partnering a try, not someone you have to try to convince. Carefully choose someone you care about and enjoy touching, learning from, and teaching.

The postures are easier if you are relatively close in height and weight, but only the friendship is essential, the physical details may vary widely. At first you may be shy, but self-consciousness will disappear as you begin to explore the ways in which your body can help your friend stretch, hold the pose, or become more comfortable in the posture. As your awareness increases, you will become sensitive to your partner's response to your touch. You will instinctively learn when to be firm or gentle, how to apply pressure, and when to release. Every awareness gained can then be taught to your friend. And just as you learn to teach your friend, you learn also to be receptive to what your friend teaches you. This balance is called Yoga.

This book is meant to be an introduction to Yoga with a friend. Try the beginning postures first, and gradually progress to the more intermediate variations. As you work together allow each other the opportunity to be inventive, and new forms will naturally evolve from the energy moving through connected bodies. Together, working unselfconsciously and with humor, you will spontaneously create postures which are just right for each of you.

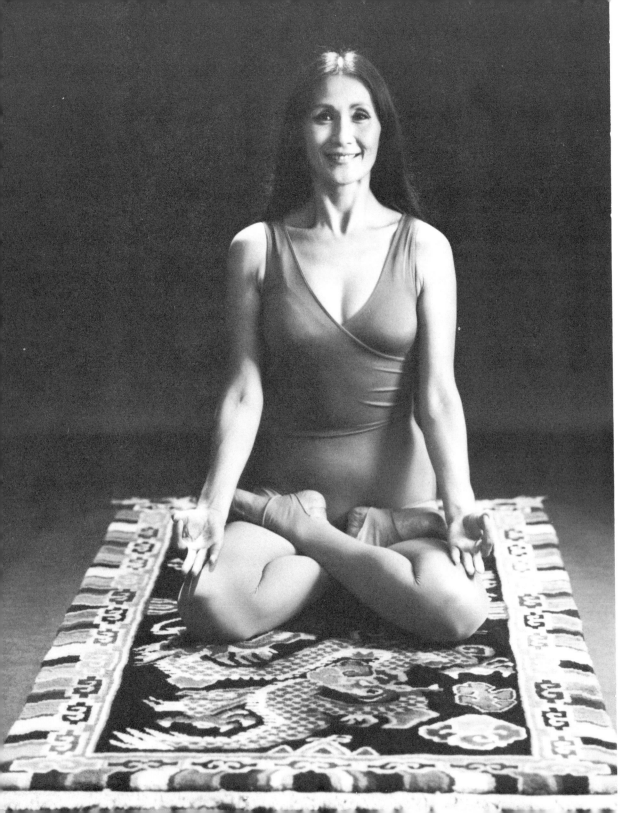

THE PARTNERS

AEJA LEE, sitting in the Full Lotus Pose (Padmasana)

Born in Korea, living in Hawaii, Aeja was schooled in Classical Korean Dance as a child. She came to Yoga to stretch, to learn to relax, and to develop a quiet mind. She especially enjoys practicing Yoga with her friends.

GLENN KAWANA, sitting in the Warrior's Pose (Virasana)

Born in Hawaii, Glenn swims, plays jazz piano, and enjoys experimenting with all aspects of Yoga. He is now in San Francisco studying to become a teacher of Yoga.

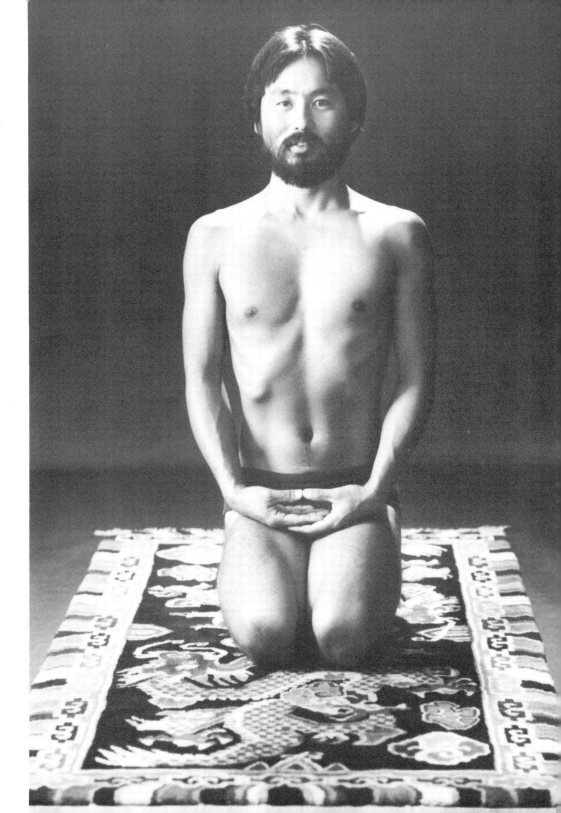

SITTING POSTURES

Without chairs, sitting is not much fun. It takes time and patience to enjoy sitting cross-legged on the floor. Yet sitting on the floor has its benefits and having a friend around for support helps.

Sitting back to back with a friend is certainly more hospitable than leaning against a wall. Plus a friend feels warm and pliable and can even be talked to.

Sitting together back to back in silence is best of all. You are alone but not lonely. Your friend can keep you quiet company without disturbing your inner thoughts. Quiet companionship is one of the joys of life.

The partners in this section are only doing one basic sitting posture, the Butterfly, with four variations. Other sitting postures, like the Lotus, are too difficult to begin with, plus they tend to hurt. In addition, the Butterfly and its variations are fun and once mastered help prepare you for other sitting poses.

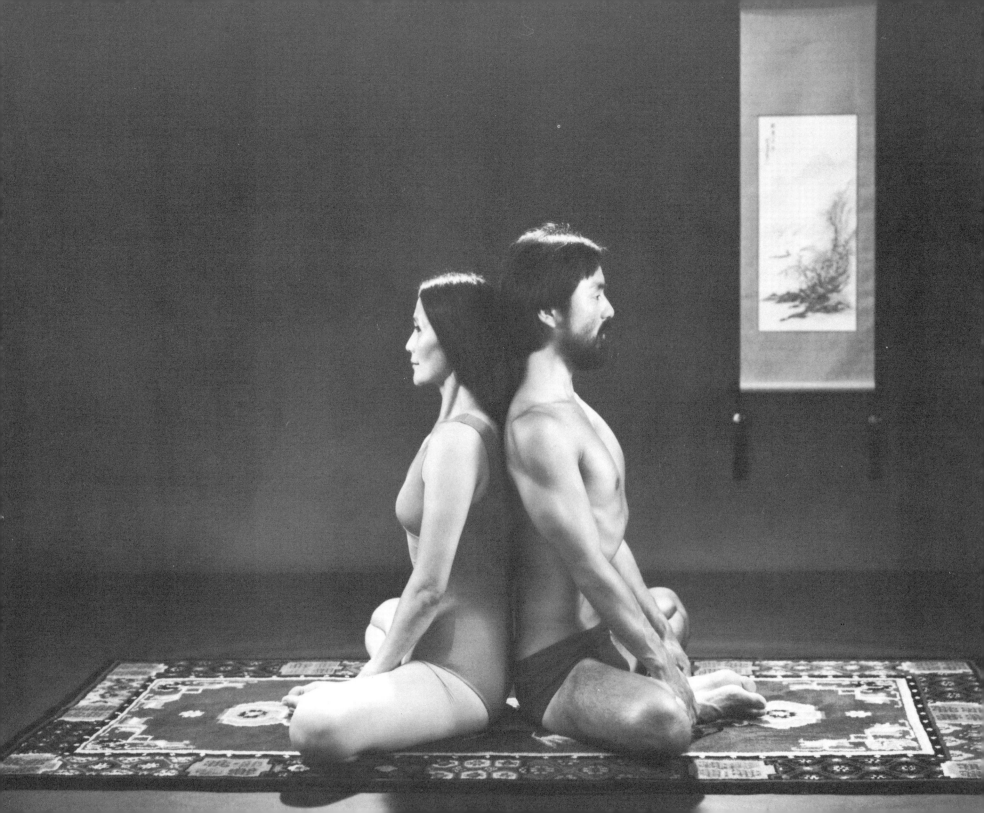

BUTTERFLY I (Baddha Konasana I)

BEGINNING POSTURE: Suitable for all students.

BENEFITS: This pose relaxes and opens the hip joints and brings a feeling of peace and relaxation to the body.

TECHNIQUE:
1. Sit back to back in the center of a blanket or rug.
2. Bring the soles of your feet together and, holding the ankles, draw your feet in as close as feels comfortable.
3. While inhaling, lift the top of your chest and feel your spine straighten and elongate. Breathe naturally.
4. Press gently into your partner's back, feeling supported from the base of the spine to the back of the head.
5. Keep the spine straight, but soften into the pose. Close your eyes and feel the warm, gentle support of your friend's back against yours. Remain together in silence for a few minutes.

"Be so silent that you hear the sound within."
B.K.S. Iyengar, SPARKS OF DIVINITY

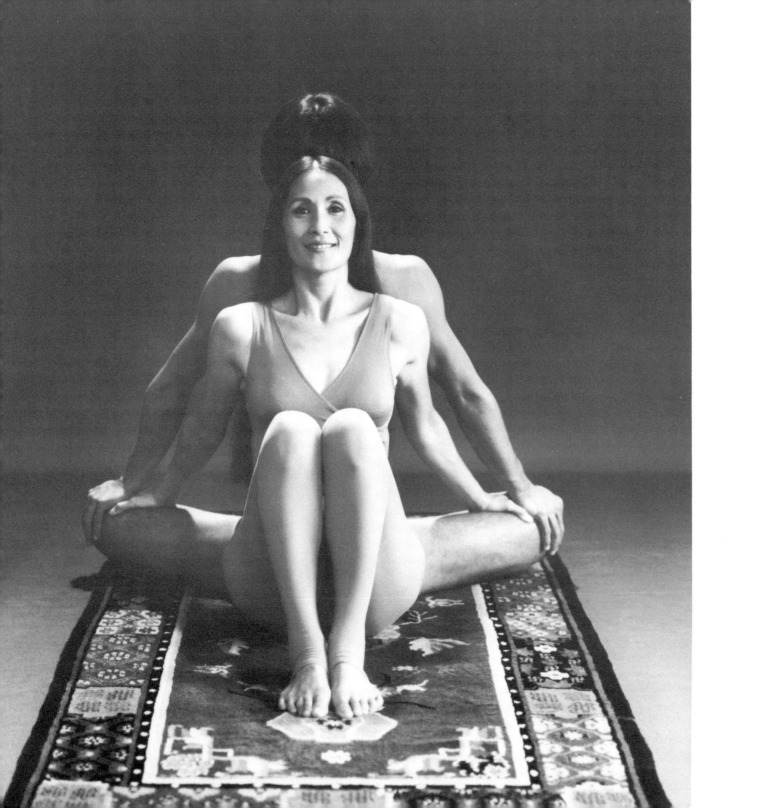

BUTTERFLY I (Baddha Konasana I) Variation

BEGINNING POSTURE: Appropriate for all students.

BENEFITS: This posture aids in relieving tightness in the hip joints by applying gentle pressure to the thighs.

TECHNIQUE:
1. Allow your partner to sit comfortably in the center of a rug with the soles of the feet together, spine straight, and hands resting lightly on the knees.
2. Sit back to back with your friend, bend your knees, and place your feet flat on the rug.
3. Create a firm connection with your friend at the base of the spine by pushing down with your feet and elongating your spine.
4. Reach back and gently rest your hands on your partner's thighs. Close your eyes and become aware of your breath. Begin to inhale and exhale together, matching your friend's breathing pattern freely and naturally with your own.
5. Inhale together, then while exhaling slowly press your partner's thighs toward the floor. Be gentle at first sensing your friend's response. As your partner relaxes, slowly increase the pressure and hold, breathing softly together in silence.
6. Release your hands slowly, allow your partner to relax with knees together. Change places and reverse the pose.

"Feeling is the eye."
  B.K.S. Iyengar, SPARKS OF DIVINITY

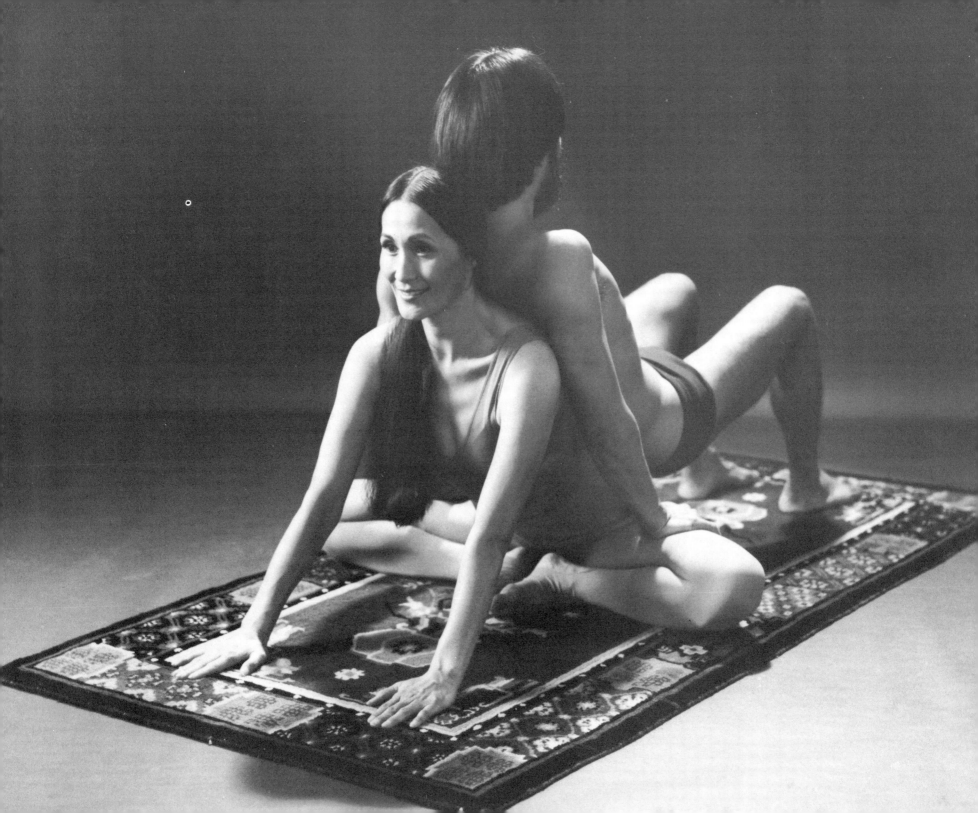

BUTTERFLY II (Baddha Konasana II)

INTERMEDIATE POSE: Suitable for students with a wide range of movement in the hip and knee joints.

BENEFITS: This pose increases the blood supply to the abdominal organs and increases the outward rotation of the hips and inward flexion of the knees.

TECHNIQUE:
1. Sit back to back in the center of a rug, bring the soles of the feet together close to the body, interlock the fingers around the feet and press the toes together.
2. While inhaling lift the top of your chest and feel your spine straighten and elongate. Hold and breathe freely.
3. Lift knees from floor, place feet on floor, put hands beside hips and lift body slightly so that your back rests firmly on your partner's, and lower your hands to your friend's thighs.
4. While exhaling, allow your friend to inch forward with straight arms, weight supported on palms.
5. Inhale and lift chest, exhale and lengthen spine, walk hands forward. Hold and breathe naturally.
6. Move as one person. As your friend stretches forward, lean back keeping the connection constant.
7. Release slowly, and reverse the posture.

"Feel the consciousness of each person as your own consciousness. So, leaving aside concern for self, become each being."
Paul Reps, "Centering," ZEN FLESH, ZEN BONES

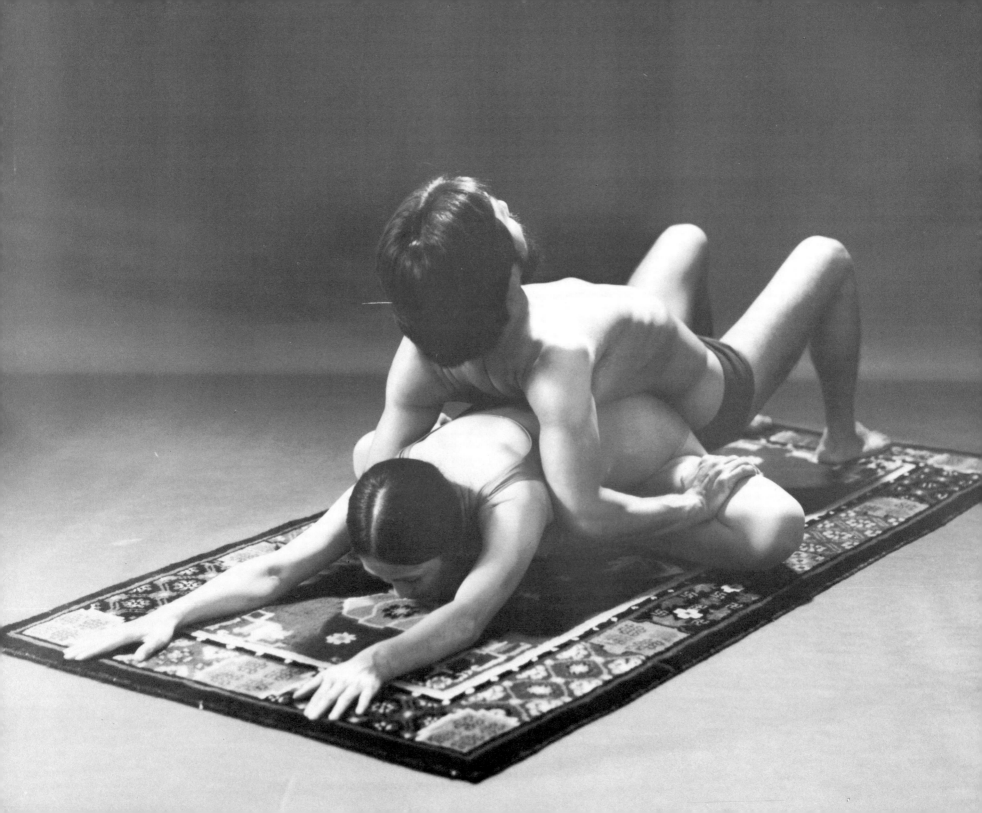

BUTTERFLY III (Baddha Konasana III)

ADVANCED POSE: Appropriate for students with excellent outward rotation of the hips, inward flexion of the knees, and forward flexibility of the spine.

BENEFITS: This pose increases the supply of blood to the abdomen, stimulating the internal organs and keeping the kidneys and bladder healthy.

TECHNIQUE:
1. Let your partner begin in the center of a rug, soles of the feet together close to the body, spine erect, hands clasping feet.
2. Release feet, walk hands forward, lift chest on an inhalation, extend spine on an exhalation. When the maximum forward movement is reached, hold, relax and breathe naturally.
3. Gently lie on your friend's back, place your hands on your partner's thighs rotating them toward your feet.
4. When your friend has accepted your weight and wishes to stretch further forward, place your upper arms against the side of your partner's ribs. Inhale together, exhale and stretch your friend gently forward.
5. Release slowly, lift body gradually, sit back to back and relax.
6. Release legs carefully, extending them completely forward, flex feet and straighten knees.
7. Rest briefly and reverse the pose.

"When you feel that you have attained the maximum stretch go beyond it. Break the barrier and go further."
B.K.S. Iyengar, BODY THE SHRINE, YOGA THY LIGHT

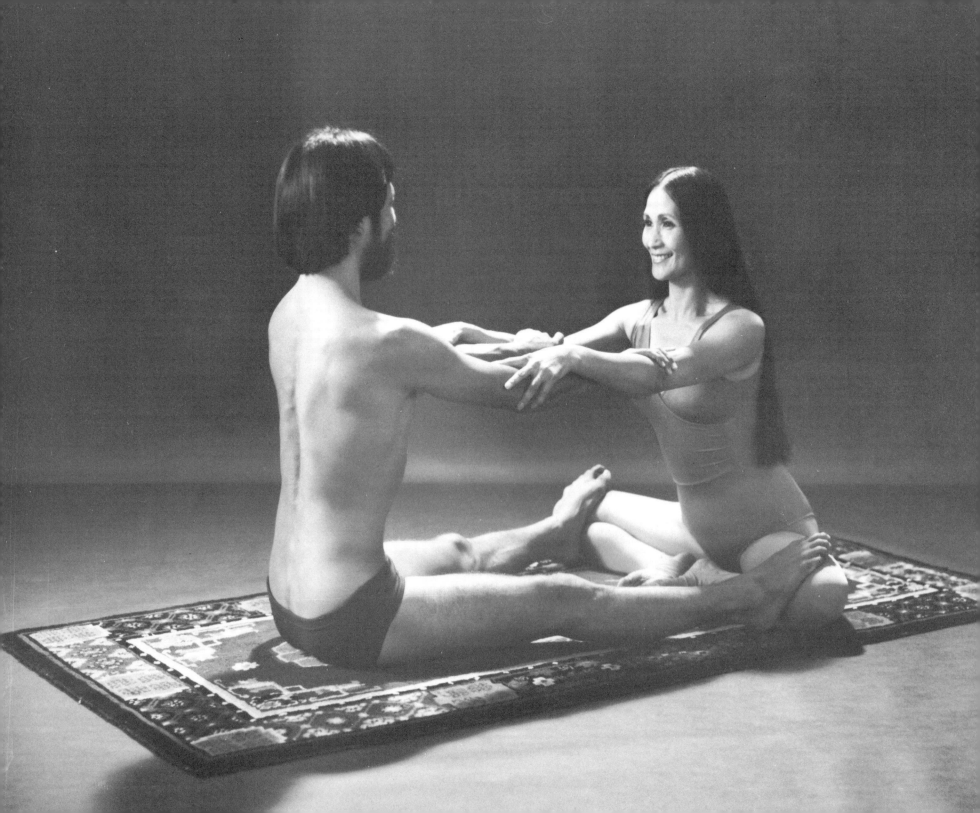

BUTTERFLY II (Baddha Konasana II) Variation

INTERMEDIATE POSE: Recommended for students who are able to sit comfortably erect with the soles of the feet together.

BENEFITS: Promotes flexibility in the hip joints and creates proper elongation and alignment of the spine.

TECHNIQUE:
1. Sit on a rug a comfortable distance apart facing each other.
2. With soles of the feet together close to the body, inhale and lift the chest, exhale and relax the inner thighs.
3. Encourage your friend to rotate the hips forward and lift and lengthen the spine before reaching forward and holding your arms wherever comfortable.
4. Place your feet gently on your partner's thighs. Exhale and press slowly toward the floor.
5. Inhale together and extend the spine, exhale and gradually ease your partner forward.
6. Look into your partner's eyes. Move forward and press down only when your friend is enjoying the pose and able to smile.
7. Release slowly, bring the knees together, and reverse the pose.

''Friends are people who help you be more yourself, more the person you are intended to be, and it is possible that without them we don't recognize ourselves, or grow to be what it is in us to be.''
Merle Shain, WHEN LOVERS ARE FRIENDS

FORWARD BENDING POSTURES

Forward bends have a reputation of being difficult, painful, and just plain hard work. The parks are filled with runners striving to stretch out by trying to bounce forward and touch their head to their knees without bending their legs.

The image of forward bends needs a change. The focus must be altered from outward to inward. Up to now the attention has been on the extremities – how to touch the hands to the feet, and the head to the knees. Creating a new image of forward bends involves changing the focus and centering the attention deep within the body.

Wherever the attention is placed will determine the effectiveness of the postures. To improve the poses create a correct base, divert your attention from the periphery and bring your awareness to the inner core of the body.

Forward bending postures originate in the hip area. When beginning concentrate on rotating the hips forward, feel the lower back become concave, the vertebrae sink deep within the spine, and all strain disappear from the back. To enjoy the poses remember to extend outward from the center and to lift and elongate the spine before moving forward.

Whenever you work forward bends with a friend the idea of extending outward from the center becomes clear. With your friend's support you experience your spine lengthening and feel the inner expansion. As the body opens outward you begin to realize that all inspiration, all awareness comes from within. Expansion is natural and friends, like flowers, open from inside out.

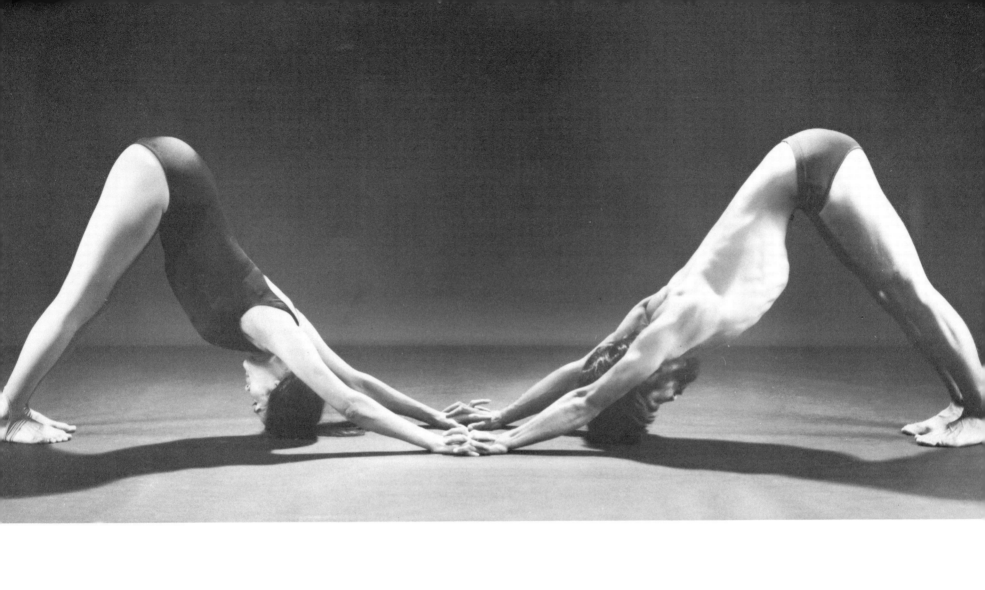

DOUBLE DOWNWARD DOG POSTURE
(Adho Mukha Svanasana)

BEGINNING POSE: Suitable for all students. Recommended especially for runners.

BENEFITS: *By increasing the blood supply to the brain, this pose helps to remove fatigue and to invigorate the body. This posture creates flexibility in the shoulders and relieves arthritis of the shoulder joints. Before running the dog pose stretches the legs, after running it relieves leg pain and brings back lost energy.*

TECHNIQUE:
1. Sit on your heels about three feet apart facing your partner.
2. Extend and straighten your arms, interlock your fingers, and place palms flat on the floor shoulder distance apart.
3. Sit back on heels, touch forehead to floor, and straighten arms.
4. Come up on all fours, curl your toes under, inhale as you raise your hips high, straighten your legs and stay high on toes.
5. Exhale, push firmly against your friend's hands and lower the head inward toward the feet, keeping the elbows straight and lengthening the spine.
6. Inhale, and while exhaling lower the heels toward the floor.
7. Hold the pose in silence, breathe freely, and feel your body extending and your mind expanding.
8. To release bend your knees, sit back on your heels, free your hands, touch your forehead to the floor and relax.

''Therefore, it is necessary to expand awareness out of the realm of inner dialogue, to loosen and open up as much as we can, and to become very silent.''
Tarthang Tulku, GESTURE OF BALANCE

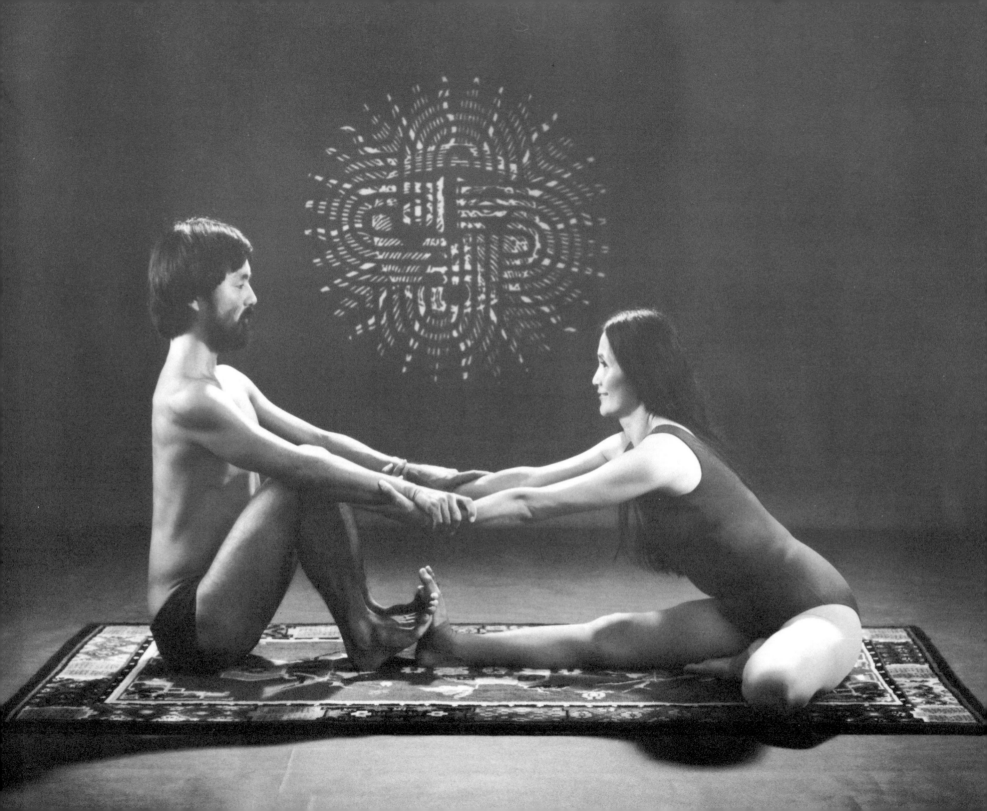

BENT LEG FORWARD BEND POSE I (Janu Sirsasana I)

BEGINNING POSTURE: Recommended for students who are able to sit with straight legs stretched outward, feet flexed, and spine erect and extended upward.

BENEFITS: This pose stretches the hamstring muscles and limbers the spine.

TECHNIQUE:

1. Sit erect facing each other, soles of the flexed feet pressed together, palms beside hips, elbows straight.
2. In unison inhale, press down with the palms and extend the spine; exhale and retain the lift.
3. Allow your partner to bend the left knee and place the left heel against the inner side of the left thigh close to the body.
4. Bend your knees and firmly support the flexed foot of your friend's extended right leg.
5. Inhale and lift the chest; exhale and clasp hands, arms straight.
6. Slowly draw your friend slightly forward. Check that the spine remains straight and the back of the knee is pressing down firmly.
7. Hold, smile at your friend, and release when ready. Change legs and repeat.
8. Relax and reverse the posture.

''Never be impatient, never discouraged, always concentrate, always realize that whatever you do is more than you did a week ago, a month ago, or even yesterday. It is progress we are concerned with.''
Jess Stearn, YOGA, YOUTH, AND REINCARNATION

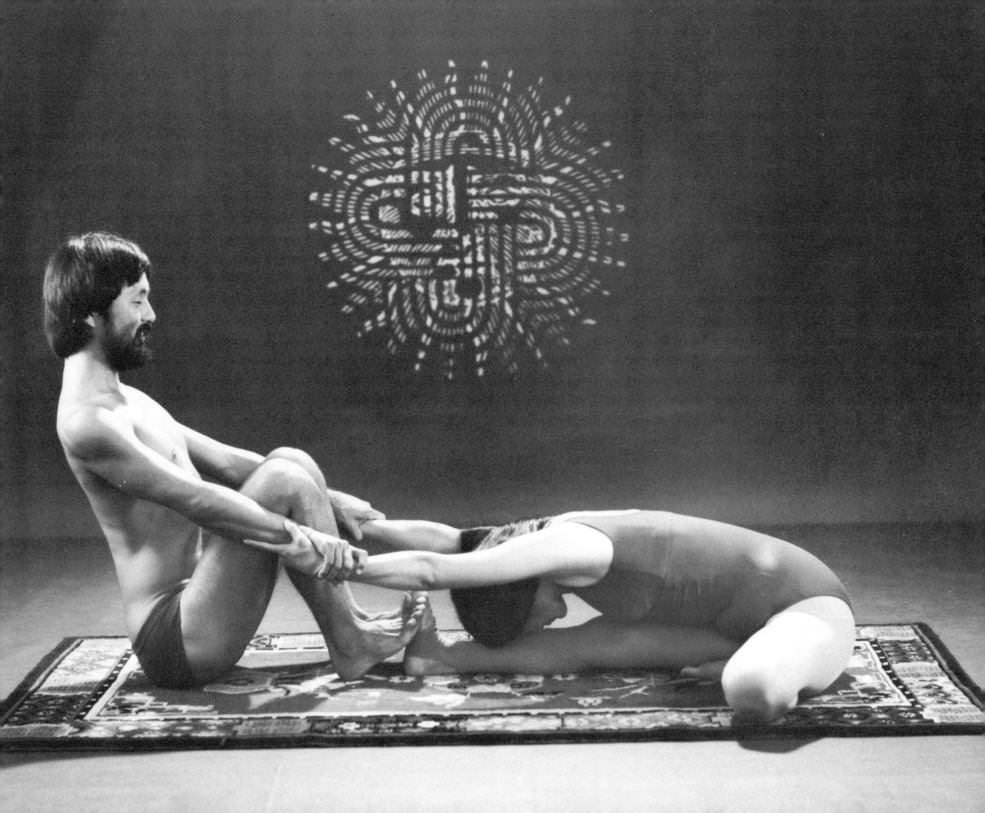

BENT LEG FORWARD BEND POSE II (Janu Sirsasana II)

INTERMEDIATE POSE: Appropriate for students with a flexible spine and stretched-out hamstring muscles.

BENEFITS: Elongates the entire spine, increases the circulation of blood to the abdomen, aids digestion and keeps the abdominal organs firm and healthy.

TECHNIQUE:
1. Sit erect facing each other, soles of the feet pressed together, spine straight.
2. Let your friend begin by drawing in the left leg and placing the left heel against the inner side of the left thigh close to the body.
3. Bend your knees and firmly support the flexed foot of your friend's extended right leg.
4. Inhale and lift the chest, exhale and clasp your partner's wrists, holding tightly and keeping your arms straight.
5. Inhale lift, exhale pull your friend forward. Continue drawing forward until the maximum stretch is reached. Hold, relax neck and abdomen, breathe freely, and allow the body and the mind to become quiet.
6. Release slowly and change legs.
7. Rest briefly and reverse the pose.

''You see more then all of your energy runs in the same direction. Concentration produces joy, so we look for things that will quiet the mind.''
Adam Smith, POWERS OF MIND

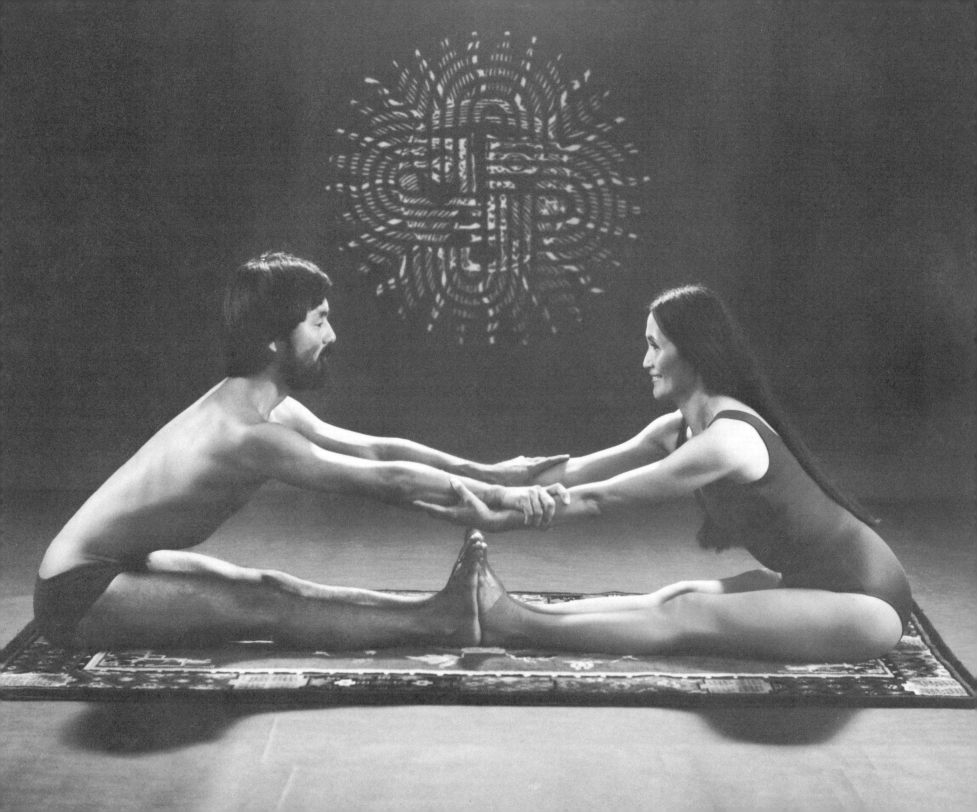

STRAIGHT LEG FORWARD BEND POSE I
(Paschimottanasana I)

BEGINNING POSE: Suitable for students who are able to sit erect and hold onto toes keeping legs straight and back flat.

BENEFITS: *Teaches correct elongation of the spine, stretches hamstring muscles, and strengthens leg muscles.*

TECHNIQUE:
1. Sit facing your friend in the center of the rug, soles of the feet firmly touching.
2. Place your palms flat beside your hips, fingers facing forward, inhale press down with palms, rotate hips forward and lift spine, exhale and hold.
3. Place hands on knees, inhale elongate spine, exhale concave the spine and advance hands toward feet. Keep the back flat.
4. Hold hands above your feet. Inhale together and lift chest, exhale and lengthen spine. Relax the abdomen and find a comfortable position to hold.
5. If one partner cannot come as far forward as the other, lift up and pull the more flexible one further forward.
6. As your bodies accustom themselves to the stretch, you and your friend may wish to increase the intensity of the movement by holding each other's wrists or forearms.
7. Release the hands, place palms on knees and push up slowly. Bend knees and relax.

''To be free we must be comfortable in being someone, anyone or no one at any time in any place.''
   A. Sujata, BEGINNING TO SEE

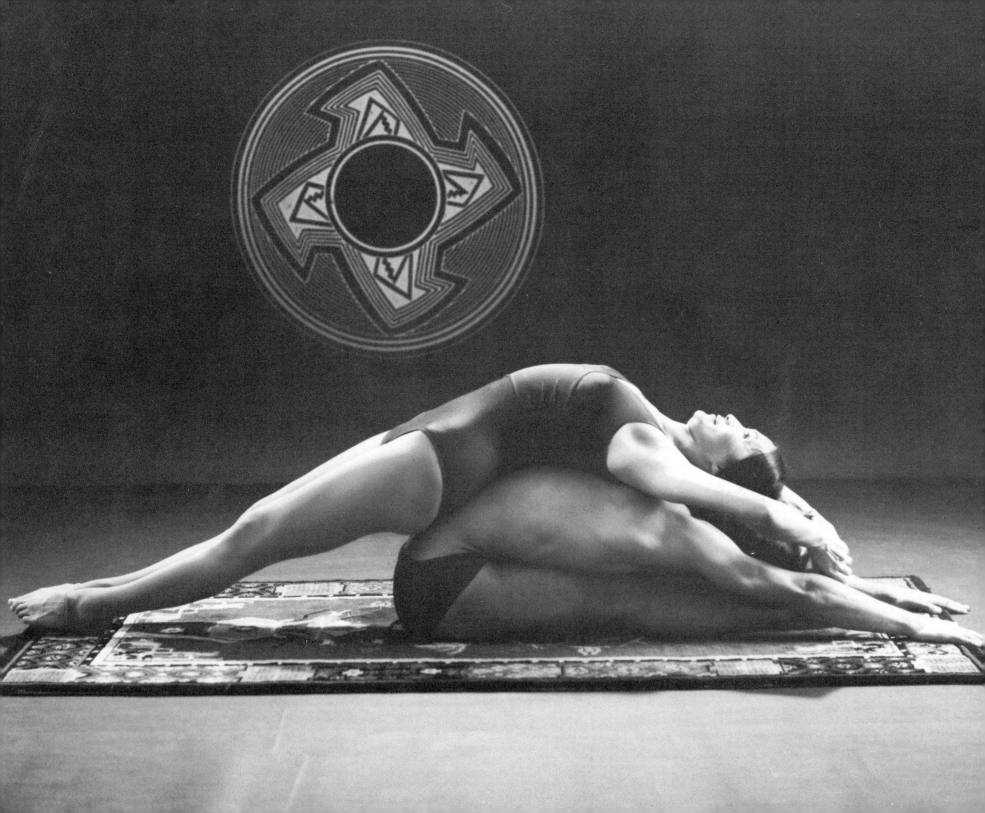

STRAIGHT LEG FORWARD BEND POSE II
(Paschimottanasana II)

BEGINNING POSE: Appropriate for students who are able to sit erect, legs straight, feet flexed, spine elongated.

BENEFITS: *Helps the spine elongate by supporting the lower back, massages the abdominal organs and improves digestion.*

TECHNIQUE:
1. Have your partner begin by sitting in the center of the rug, hips rotated forward, legs straight, feet flexed.
2. Inhale lift chest, extend the spine from the hips, exhale and move forward, reach out and hold legs, ankles, or feet.
3. Continue to advance forward until the maximum extension is reached. Hold, relax the abdomen and breathe freely.
4. Carefully place your lower back in contact with your friend's lower back. Supporting your partner's lower back firmly, encourage your friend to inhale and pull the chest forward, and then to exhale completely.
5. If your friend is comfortable in the pose you may lie down on your partner's back, extend your legs, and reach back and hold your friend's feet.
6. Soften into the pose, enjoy supporting your friend, realize that your weight has enabled your friend to let go, to stretch further than ever before.
7. Release slowly, breathe deeply, and reverse the pose.

"The art of surrender is exhalation."
    B.K.S. Iyengar, SPARKS OF DIVINITY

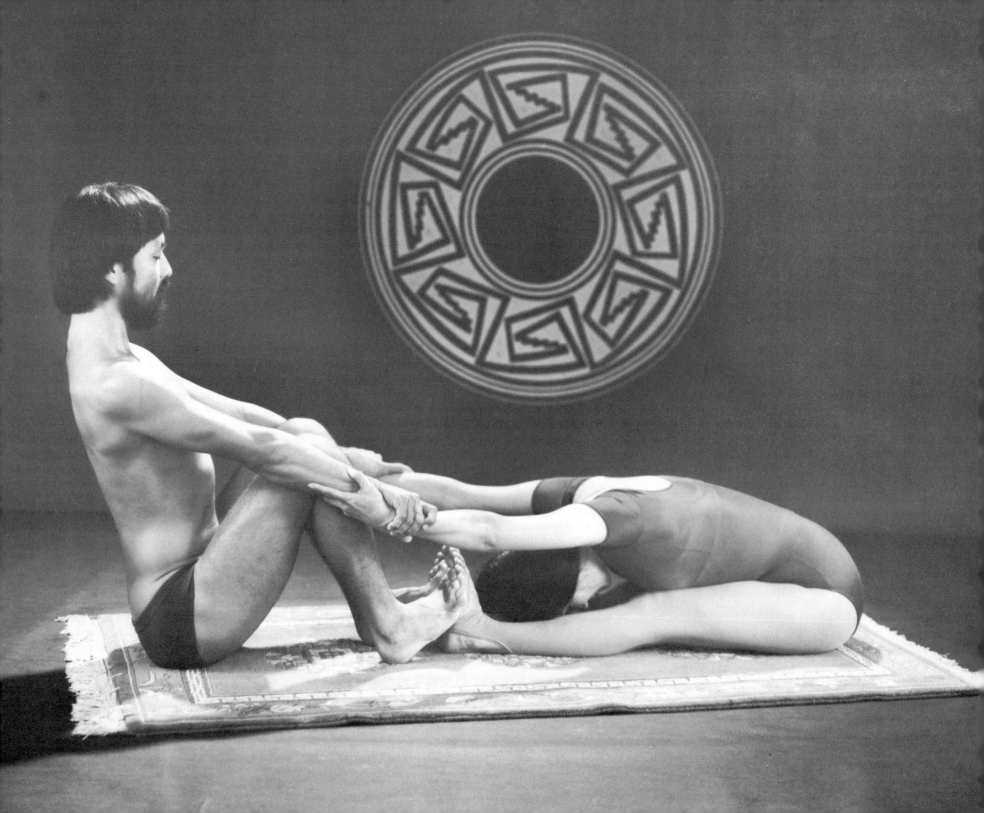

STRAIGHT LEG FORWARD BEND POSE III
(Paschimottanasana III)

INTERMEDIATE POSE: Suitable for students with a limber spine, and stretched-out leg muscles.

BENEFITS: Invigorates the entire spine and increases flexibility in the shoulders and wrists.

TECHNIQUE:
1. Sit facing your friend, knees bent. Place your feet firmly against the flexed feet of your partner's extended legs.
2. Reach forward and hold onto your partner's wrists.
3. Inhale together and lift, exhale and pull your partner forward, straighten your spine and exert steady pressure on your partner's feet.
4. Move evenly together using your hands and feet as leverage and gradually lengthen your friend's spine.
5. Breathe softly and experience an inner expansion beginning at the base of the spine and extending outward all the way to the tips of the fingers.
6. Release hands, place palms on knees and push up slowly. Bend knees to chest and hold, resting head on knees.
7. Relax and then reverse the posture.

"Think light. Try to impart a feeling of lightness to the body. This can be done by mentally extending yourself outwards from the center of your body. Do not think of yourself as a small compressed suffering thing. Think of yourself as graceful and expanding—no matter how unlikely it may seem at the time."

B.K.S. Iyengar, SPARKS OF DIVINITY

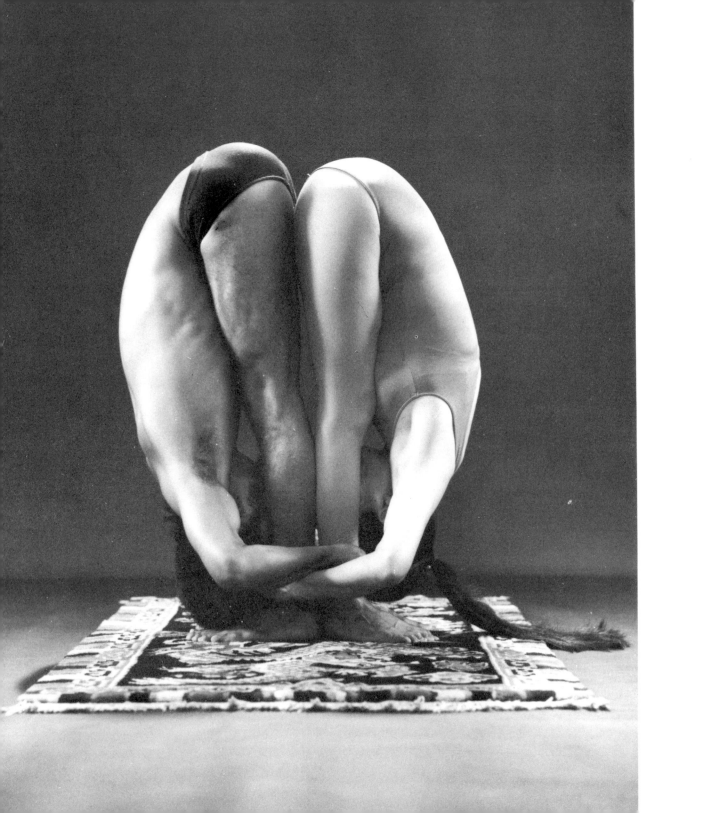

STANDING FORWARD BEND POSE (Uttanasana)

ADVANCED POSE: Appropriate for students who are able to bend forward from a standing position, place palms on the floor beside the feet, touch the chest to thighs, and straighten legs.

BENEFITS: This pose tones the abdominal organs, aids digestion, improves balance, soothes the nerves, and calms the mind.

TECHNIQUE:
1. Stand back to back about one foot apart in the center of a rug or on the floor.
2. Place hands on hips, relax abdomen, bend forward, reach out and touch palms to floor in front of feet.
3. Exhale and place palms beside feet. Bend knees slightly and walk back until legs are touching. Straighten knees, rotate hips downward, flatten palms beside feet, and press evenly against your partner's legs.
4. When you feel balanced reach back and hold onto each other's ankles. Breathe freely and relax your shoulders.
5. Feel the energy moving through connected bodies. Gradually become aware of the subtle cooperation needed to maintain the delicate balance.
6. Holding each other's ankles reach the maximum stretch by lifting the chest forward and extending the head closer to the feet.
7. To release place hands forward on floor, bend knees slightly, take a step forward, roll up, and rest in a standing position.

"You are not alone but linked to everything around you."
Janwillem van de Wetering, A GLIMPSE OF NOTHINGNESS

SIDE STRETCHES OF THE BODY AND INNER LEGS

Everyone loves to stretch. Stretching frees the body and when the body is free the mind begins to expand. Tension is trapped within the body and because the body's natural state is freedom, tension creates depression.

The secret of complete relaxation is complete extension. This means not just stretching the legs, but extending the entire body outward from the center.

Create an image of a ball of energy located deep within your abdomen. With eyes closed imagine that energy expanding in all directions, moving downward through your feet, radiating outward through your fingertips, and coursing upward through the top of your head. When that ball of energy is completely dispersed only calmness remains.

Stretching with your friend makes this image of expansion real. When all tension is gone the body quiets and the mind is at peace. The key is total stretch, the result is total relaxation.

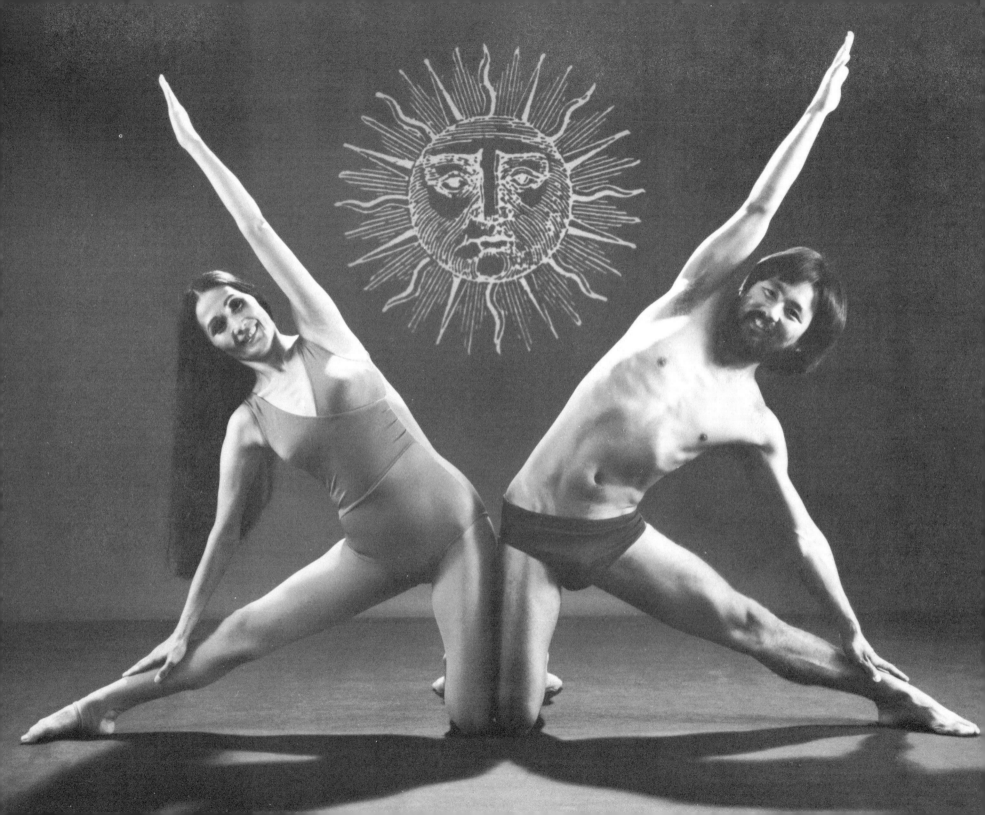

BEAM POSTURE (Parighasana)

BEGINNING POSE: A basic stretching posture for all students.

BENEFITS: This pose helps to relieve stiffness in the back, and aids in keeping the abdominal muscles and organs in good condition.

TECHNIQUE:
1. Kneel in the center of the mat with the outside of your left thigh touching your partner's right thigh.
2. Extend the opposite leg out to the side, toes pointing, with the outside of the foot firmly on the floor. Keep the hips level and facing the front.
3. Raise your arms and extend them upward. Supported by your friend, stretch upward together.
4. Inhale together, and while exhaling, slide your inside hips toward each other. Reaching out, extend the upper body away from the center, and then lower the outside arm, resting the hand on the top of the shin.
5. Hold this pose, breathing freely, and firmly supporting your friend. Extend your inner arm upward. Create a straight line, resembling a bar or beam, from your hipbone to your fingertips.
6. Exhale, straighten up, and reverse the posture.

"Relaxation follows extension."
  B.K.S. Iyengar, SPARKS OF DIVINITY

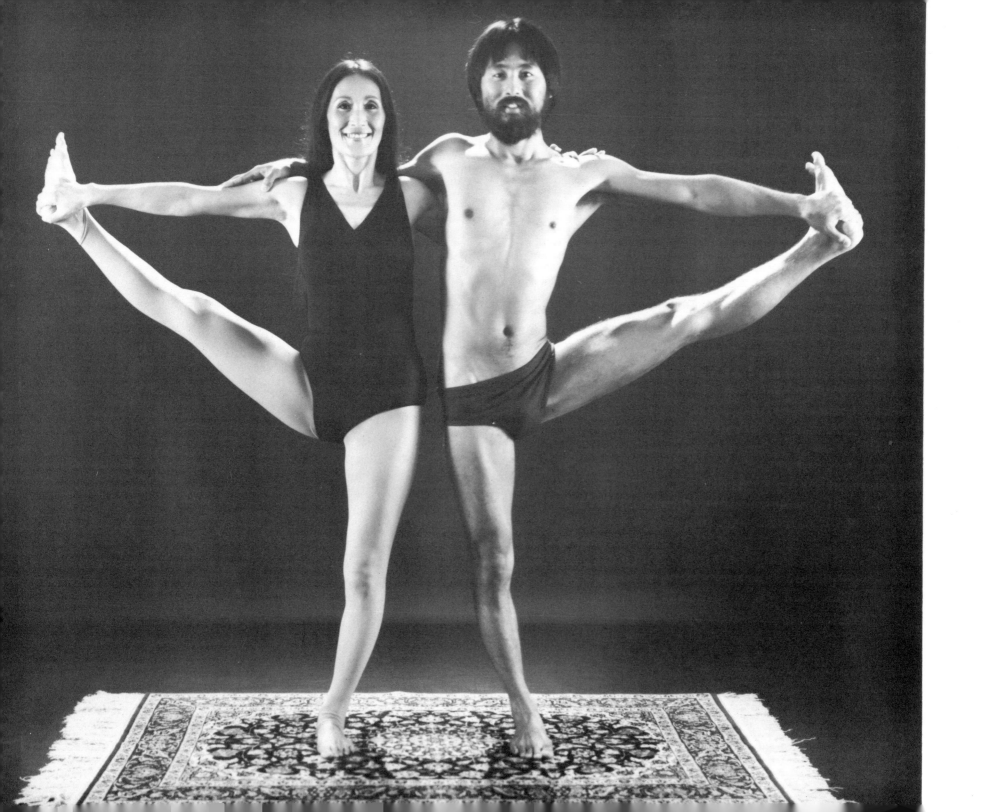

STANDING LEG STRETCH (Utthita Padangustasana)

INTERMEDIATE POSE: Suggested for students who are able to stand on one leg, extend the other leg to the side, hold onto ankle, big toe, or arch of foot, and keep the chest lifted and spine erect.

BENEFITS: Stretches and strengthens the leg muscles, improves balance, and increases flexibility in the hip joints.

TECHNIQUE:

1. Stand side by side with your friend a few inches apart, feet together, arms resting by your sides.
2. Close your eyes and concentrate on extending mentally outward from your center, lifting and elongating your spine and stretching and tightening your legs. Slowly open your eyes.
3. When your base is firm place your inside arm securely around your friend's shoulders.
4. Inhale together and bend outside knee bringing it close to chest. Reach down the inside of the leg and take hold of the big toe of the bent leg.
5. Exhale and straighten the leg in front of you. If the leg is still bent hold the ankle instead. You may also prefer holding the inside arch of the foot.
6. When your balance is stable, move the leg around to the side, hold, extend outward and breathe freely.
7. Slowly release, bend knee and lower foot to the floor. Change places and reverse the leg.

''The essence of communication is intention.''
Werner Erhard, IF GOD HAD MEANT MAN TO FLY HE WOULD HAVE GIVEN HIM WINGS

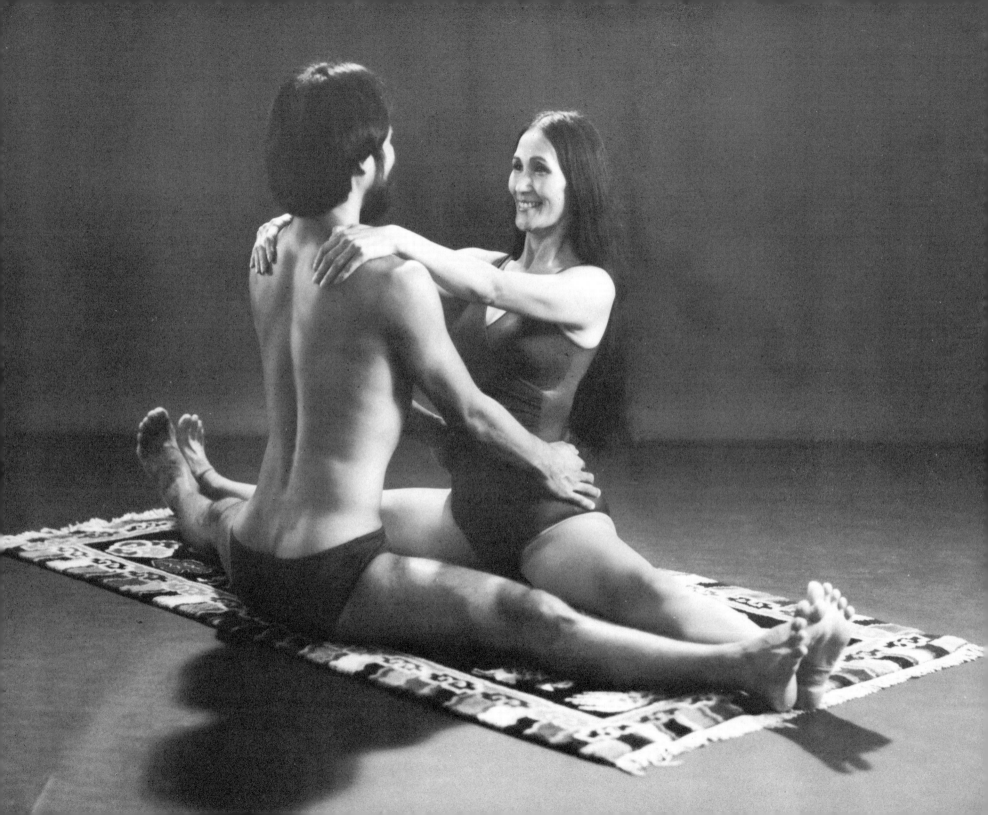

WIDE ANGLE LEG STRETCH (Konasana)

BEGINNING POSE: Suitable for all students.

BENEFITS: Stretches the inner thigh muscles, helps improve posture.

TECHNIQUE:
1. Sit facing your friend on a rug, legs spread apart, feet or ankles touching. Widen your legs a comfortable distance apart, and extend the heels to straighten the legs.
2. Place your hands on the floor directly behind you, fingers pointing away. Inhale together, and while exhaling push with the fingers rotating the hips forward and concaving the spine.
3. Exert gentle, steady pressure on each other's legs. Continue to lift, rotate forward, and widen legs until maximum stretch is reached.
4. When spine is straight release hands, place your hands on your friend's hips and rotate the hips forward.
5. Let your partner's hands rest lightly on your shoulders. Hold in silent communication and then change hand positions.
6. Release by moving backward on the rug, lifting the knees together close to the chest, place feet flat, and relax forward resting head on knees.

''The only wealth that really counts is having loving friends.''
Merle Shain, WHEN LOVERS ARE FRIENDS

BACKBENDING POSTURES

All backward bending is a step into the unknown. Our bodies, like the moon, have a light and a dark side. We see the front side of our body all the time – it is familiar, it is the home of our heart and of our breath. Relying almost exclusively on our sense of sight, we ignore our back because we cannot see it. Our back remains the unknown part of our body, its shell, the part we expose to the world while instinctively protecting our front side from harm.

Whenever there is something about our body or our life which we cannot see or understand, that insecurity becomes a source of fear. When we learn to dive we usually learn a front dive first. Then only as our confidence grows do we attempt a back dive.

It is the same with Yoga. As we learn to arch the spine backward, to eventually push up into a backbend from the floor, only then do we begin to conquer this fear of the unknown. Anytime we face our fear, go further than we did before, the anxiety begins to recede and we become aware of a new feeling of freedom.

Tension is trapped within our spine. As we bend and stretch our spine we release that accumulated tension and with it goes depression and a feeling of lightness and joy gradually permeates our being.

Because we cannot see our back we need to become aware of our spine through a subtle inner sensitivity, an awareness of how the spine feels. As we learn to differentiate between a feeling of pain and a feeling of stretch, the fear of injuring our spine gives way to a desire for openness, for flexibility, and for release.

Knowledge gained through experiencing our spine in a variety of backbending postures helps relieve chronic back pain and creates a feeling of youth and vitality. As we identify the source of pain and tightness, learn how to protect the spine by tightening the buttocks and extending from the chest, we gain confidence in our body and know its actual limits.

Once we have experienced change, have stretched further, have exceeded an old pain boundary, and have discovered something of value for ourselves, this feeling of achievement is ours alone.

We have all seen very old people walking slowly with backs hunched, leaning forward with rounded shoulders and withdrawing their participation from the world. One way to reenter life, at any age, is to continually expand the chest, roll back the shoulders, and gracefully arch the spine. After a while with consistent practice the spine regains its lost flexibility. Then, no longer strapped by a stiff, unyielding body, we regain our lost movement and, lithe as a cat, become free to be whatever we want to be.

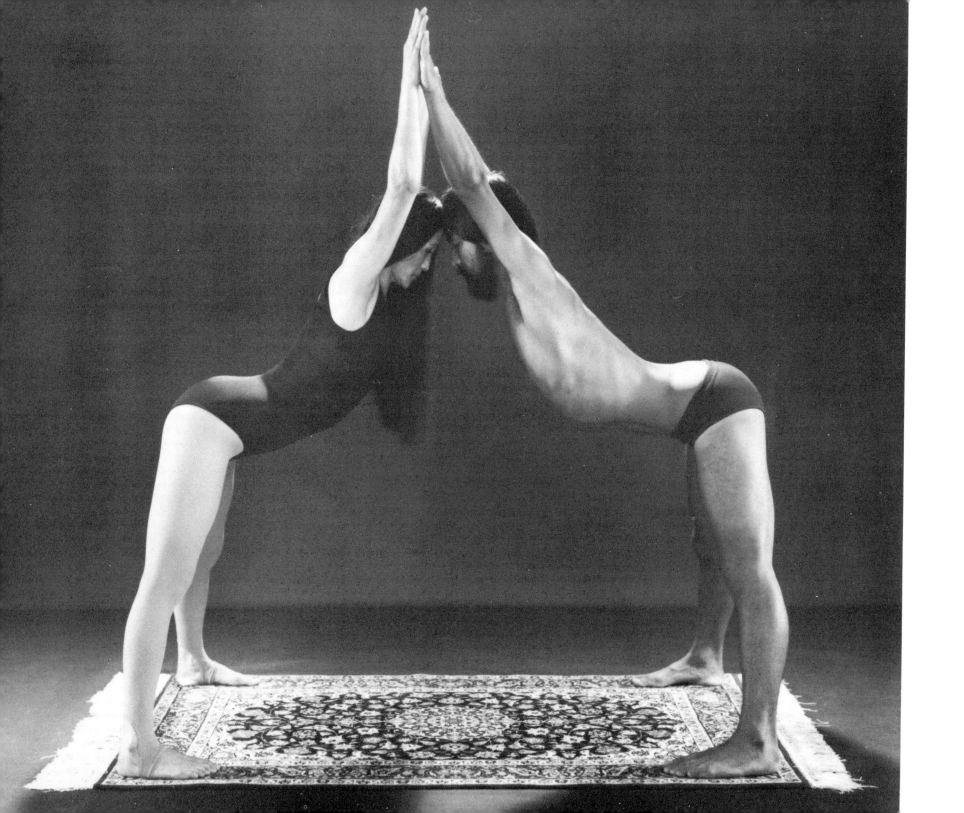

CHEST EXPANSION POSTURE (Prasarita Padottanasana)

BEGINNING POSE: Suitable for all students.

BENEFITS: This posture stretches the hamstring muscles of the legs, evenly elongates the entire spine, and increases flexibility in the shoulders.

TECHNIQUE:
1. Stand facing your partner about four feet away on a non-skid floor or rug.
2. Widen your legs three to four feet apart with the outside edges of the feet parallel to each other, toes turned slightly inward.
3. Inhale, tighten the legs by drawing up the kneecaps and place the hands on the hips. Exhale, bend forward, lead with lifted chest, and work to concave the lower back.
4. Release hands from hips and join hands with your friend, firmly pressing palms and fingers together, arms straight.
5. Inhale and raise hands as high as you can. Exhale, press palms together, aim buttocks backward, tighten leg muscles, and center weight evenly on the feet.
6. As you hold the pose together, create an equal stretch, touch foreheads, feel the shoulders opening, and experience an even lengthening of the entire spine.
7. Release hands slowly, weight on feet, straighten up, bring legs together, and rest in a standing position.

"We can just be. We do not need to think about 'me' or 'you' or what we are gaining or losing; we can just expand our feeling, our relaxation, our calmness, and our joy."
Tarthang Tulku, GESTURE OF BALANCE

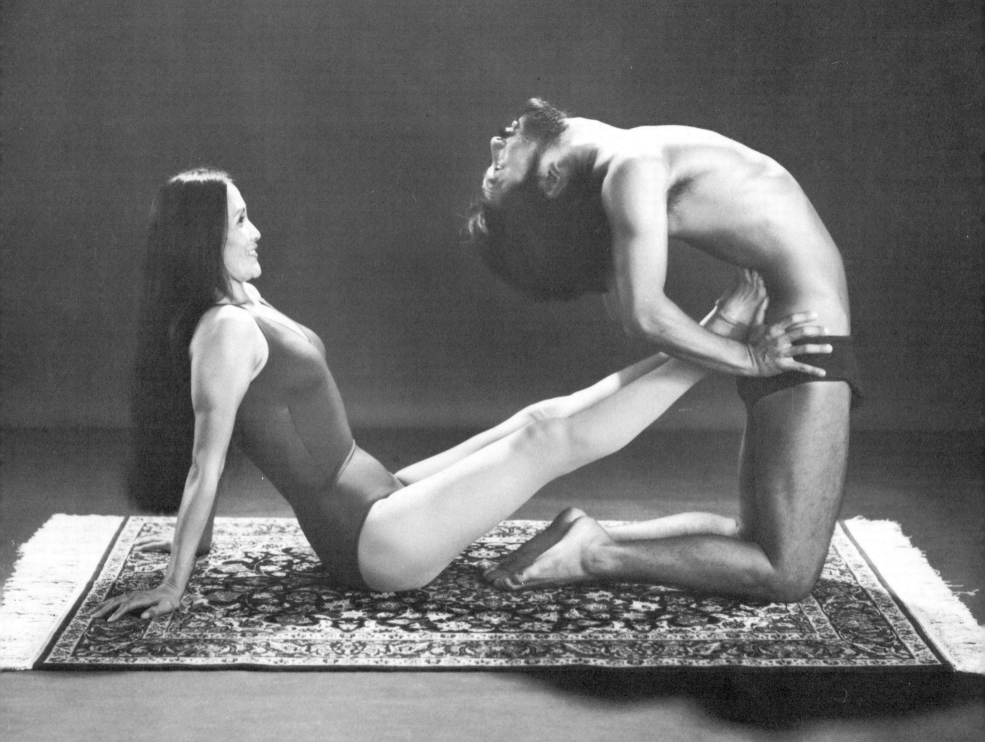

CAMEL POSTURE I (Ustrasana I)

BEGINNING POSE: Recommended for all students.

BENEFITS: This posture stretches the entire spine and the thigh muscles, strengthens the neck, and expands the chest.

TECHNIQUE:

1. Allow your partner to kneel on a rug with the knees and feet slightly apart.
2. Inhale and place the palms on the hips. Exhale and rotate the shoulders back and down bringing the elbows toward each other.
3. Inhale stretch the neck and lift the chin to the ceiling; exhale and drop the head back keeping the neck stretched and the shoulders down. Hold, breathing freely.
4. To help your friend increase the lift across the chest, sit directly behind and place your feet evenly on either side of your partner's spine. Place your palms behind you as a brace.
5. Inhaling together lift the chest; exhale and press your friend's hips forward and hold.
6. Experiment with the placement of the feet on the spine. Allow your friend to let you know where your feet offer the best support.
7. Release your feet and rest. Let your friend come up slowly, lifting the chin to the ceiling and forward with the neck stretched and shoulders lowered. Release hands, rest sitting on heels, breathing slowly and deeply.
8. Change places and reverse the posture.

"Health is a function of participation."
Werner Erhard, IF GOD HAD MEANT MAN TO FLY HE WOULD HAVE GIVEN HIM WINGS

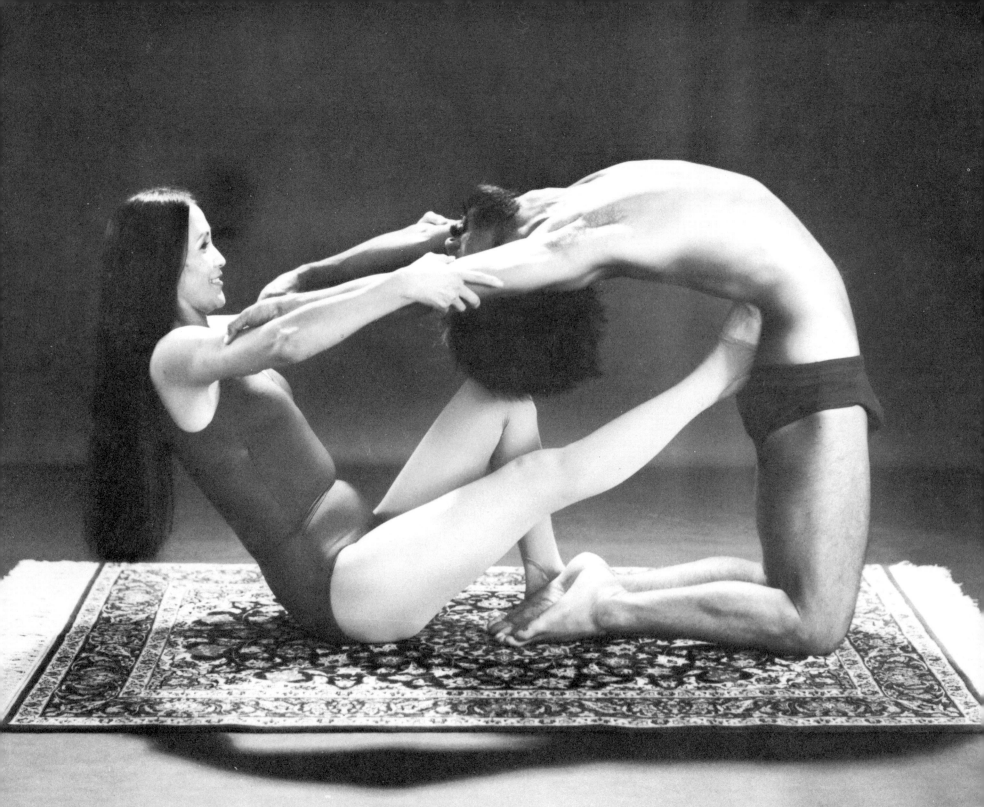

CAMEL POSTURE II (Ustrasana II)

INTERMEDIATE POSE: Suitable for students with backward flexibility of the spine and openness of the shoulders.

BENEFITS: This pose stretches the thigh muscles, elongates the entire spine, stretches the shoulder joints, and expands the chest.

TECHNIQUE:
1. Let your partner kneel on a rug, knees and feet together, hands on hips, shoulders rotated back and down, and elbows moving in toward each other.
2. Inhale stretch the neck and lift the chin, exhale and drop the head back. Push hips forward to their maximum.
3. Sit directly behind your friend, bend one knee and place the foot flat beside your partner's feet. Place the other foot in the center of your friend's lower back. Have your friend tell you where to place your foot for the most support and comfort.
4. Allow your partner to release hands from hips. Inhale, lift hands and straighten arms over head. Exhale and extend arms backward.
5. Hold your friend's arms securely. Inhale and lift chest, exhale and push firmly forward with foot while drawing arms back as far as is comfortable. Hold, breathing freely.
6. Inhale and release arms, exhale and lower arms. Come up slowly and rest sitting on your heels.
7. Change places and reverse the posture.

"Consider your essence as light rays rising from center to center up the vertebrae and so rises livingness in you."
Paul Reps, "Centering," ZEN FLESH, ZEN BONES

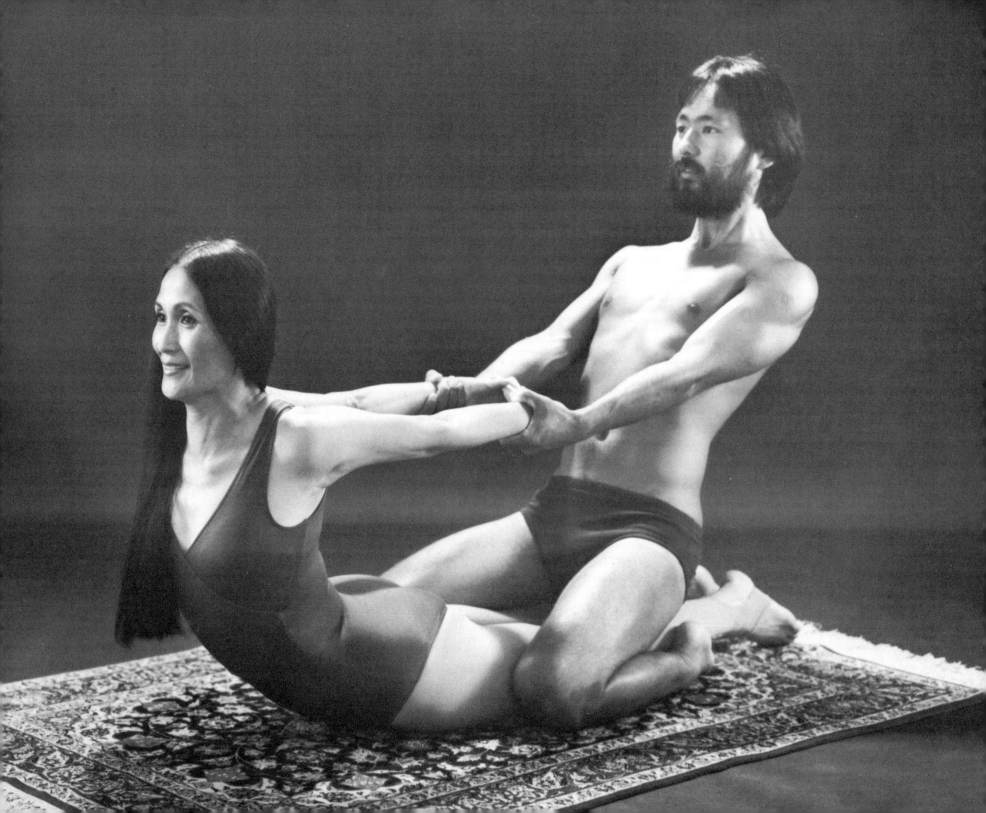

EXTENDED COBRA POSE (Bhujangasana)

BEGINNING POSE: Appropriate for all students.

BENEFITS: *This pose helps to recreate the natural curve of the spine, to realign the vertebrae, to expand the chest and stretch the shoulder joints.*

TECHNIQUE:
1. Lie face down on a rug. Lift the head, tuck in the chin, and lower the forehead to the rug.
2. Interlock your fingers tightly behind your back, press your palms together, lift your shoulders and roll them back and down feeling your arms stretch and straighten.
3. Your friend then kneels on either side of your legs and, finding a comfortable position, sits gently on your calves or ankles.
4. Tighten the buttocks muscles firmly. Inhale and lift, stretching the chest forward and up; exhale and extend the arms backward.
5. When you have reached your maximum lift on your own, your friend will grasp your wrists firmly and pull you further up and back.
6. Communicate with your friend just how far you wish to go. Stop and breathe freely. As the spine stretches, your partner may slowly draw you further back while you continue to lift your chest.
7. Close your eyes and experience from inside out this new feeling of expansion and freedom.
8. Keep buttocks tight throughout the pose to protect your lower back from strain and to enable you to stretch beyond your normal ability.
9. Slowly lower the body to the mat, relax the arms at the sides and rest. Breathe deeply and exhale fully.
10. Change places and reverse the posture.

''This feeling of expansion is much more powerful than the physical sensation of joy – it is deep, vast, infinite.''
Tarthang Tulku, GESTURE OF BALANCE

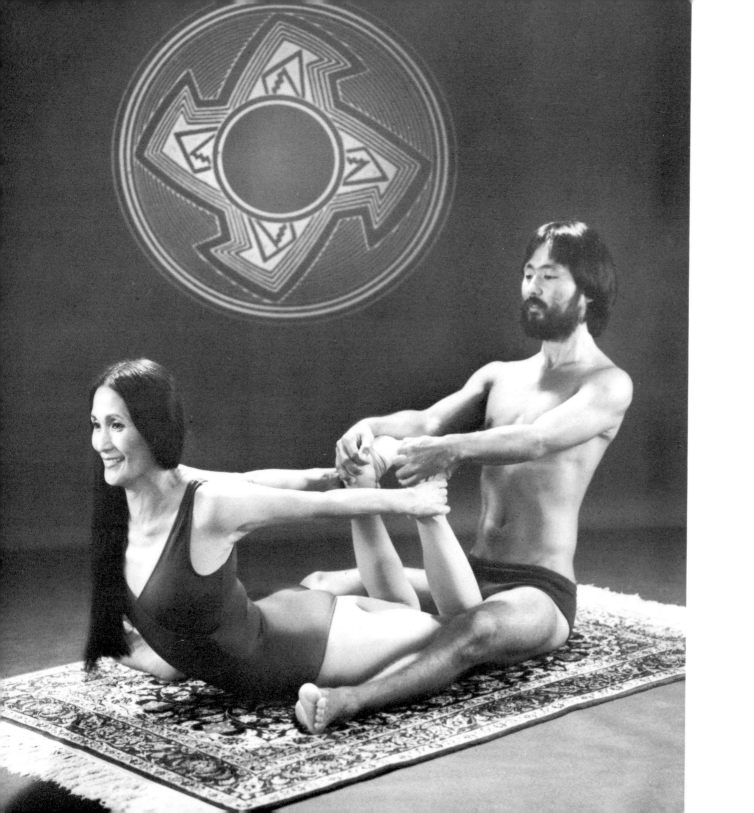

BOW POSTURE (Dhanurasana)

INTERMEDIATE POSE: Recommended for students with backward flexibility of the spine. Learn Camel and Cobra poses first.

BENEFITS: This pose strengthens and aligns the spine, tones the abdomen, and aids digestion.

TECHNIQUE:
1. Lie face down, tuck in the chin, and rest the forehead on the rug.
2. Bend the knees and take hold of the ankles from the outside. Squeeze the shoulder blades together.
3. Inhale and tighten the buttocks, exhale and lift the chest and the knees off of the floor. Stretch the neck and hold the pose, breathing freely.
4. To increase the height and the stretch of the pose, allow your friend to sit or kneel alongside your knees and hold onto your heels or your wrists.
5. Inhale together and, while exhaling, extend the chest forward and up as your friend gradually pulls your feet back. Let your partner know when you have reached your maximum stretch. Relax and hold the lift.
6. Enjoy the support of your friend and silently experience a feeling of openness in the chest area.
7. Slowly lower the legs and release the hands. Rest until your breathing has returned to normal.
8. Change places and reverse the posture.

"Your body lives in the past, your mind in the future. They come together in the present when you practice Yoga."
B.K.S. Iyengar, BODY THE SHRINE, YOGA THY LIGHT

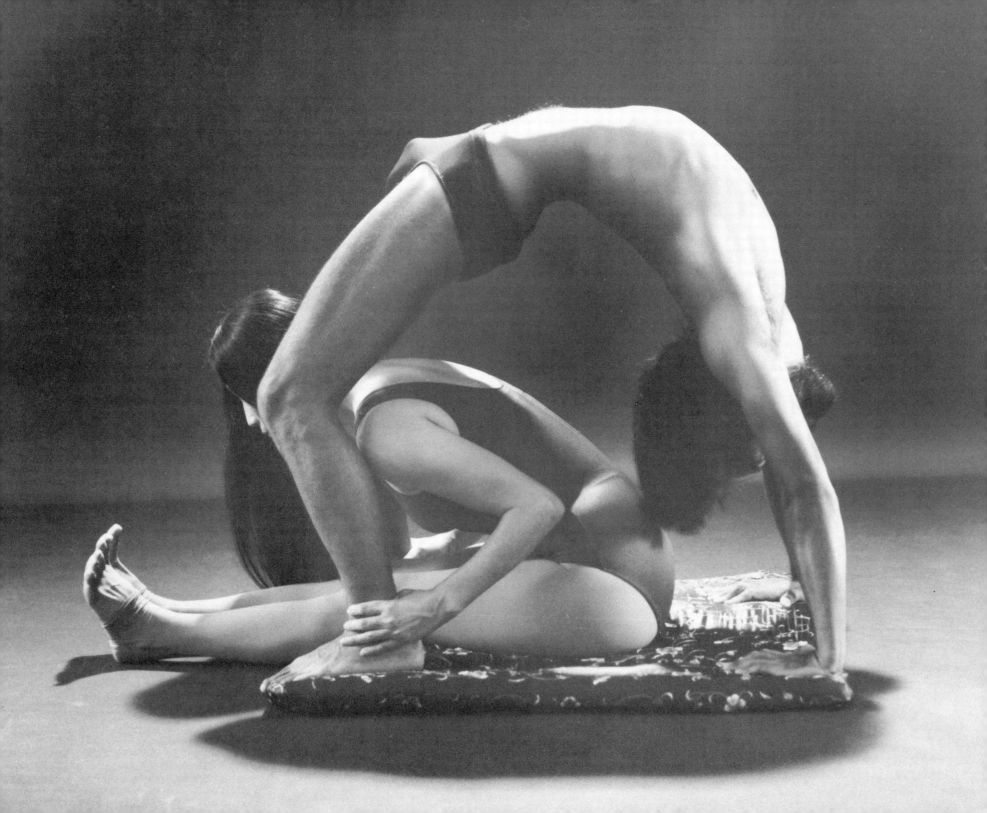

WHEEL POSTURE I (Urdhva Dhanurasana I)

INTERMEDIATE POSE: Recommended for students with strong wrists and arms, openness in the shoulder joints, and backward flexibility of the spine.

BENEFITS: This posture strengthens the arms and wrists, develops a supple spine, and brings new energy and vitality to the body.

TECHNIQUE:
1. Begin with your partner in the supported Shoulderstand position. (See page 72 for detailed instructions for the supported Shoulderstand posture.)
2. Allow your friend to release your ankles and then to place the palms flat on the rug. Extend your legs and flex your feet.
3. Your partner then bends both knees and lowers them over your shoulders.
4. Inhale together and while exhaling begin to come forward just far enough so your friend can lower both feet to the rug. Hold onto your partner's ankles firmly.
5. Inhaling, your partner places both hands, palms down, under the shoulders. While exhaling, your friend tightens the buttocks, pushes down with the palms and the feet, and then lifts the chest and straightens both arms.
6. Breathe freely and hold, continuing to expand the chest.
7. To release, your friend tucks the chin to the chest and lowers the shoulders and arms to the mat. Let go of your partner's ankles, slowly sit up, and allow your friend to lift both legs back into the Shoulderstand.
8. Move aside so your friend can slowly roll out of the Shoulderstand and rest.
9. Change places and reverse the pose.

"Be careful with your back and do the asana thoughtfully with the name of God on the lips."
B.K.S. Iyengar, SPARKS OF DIVINITY

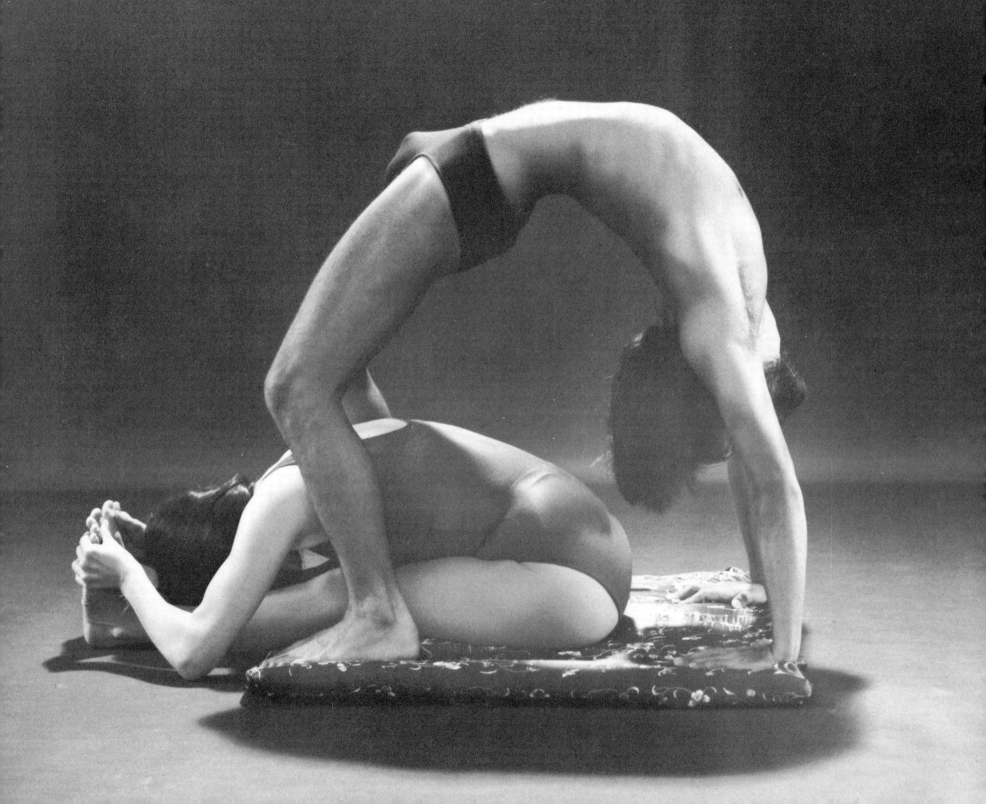

WHEEL POSTURE II (Urdhva Dhanurasana II)

ADVANCED POSE: Appropriate for students with strong arms, forward and backward flexibility of the spine, strong back muscles, stretched-out thigh muscles, and secure balance.

BENEFITS: This posture strengthens arms, legs and spine, stretches thigh muscles, and improves balance.

TECHNIQUE:
1. Begin with your partner in the supported Shoulderstand pose. (See page 72 for detailed instructions for the Shoulderstand.)
2. Let your friend release your ankles and place arms, palms down, on the rug. Extend your legs, feet flexed.
3. Your friend then bends both knees and lowers them over your shoulders.
4. Inhale together and lift your chest. Exhale and as your friend lowers both feet to the floor, reach forward and firmly grasp the sides of your feet and pull your toes back.
5. Inhaling, your partner places hands, palms down, under the shoulders. While exhaling, your friend tightens the buttocks, turns toes slightly inward, presses down with the feet and the palms, lifts high from the chest and the tailbone, and straightens the arms completely. Hold the posture and breathe naturally and freely.
6. Coordinating your movements with your partner's, inhale together and lift your chest as your friend further arches the back and extends the chest.
7. Exhale together, pull yourself forward, and let your friend help you maintain your new forward stretch by supporting your side ribs with pressure of the legs.
8. Before releasing, your friend lifts the tailbone high, tightens the buttocks, and further stretches the thighs. Then your friend tucks the chin to the

chest, lowers the arms and shoulders to the rug, and raises the legs back into the Shoulderstand as you sit up.

9. Move aside, let your friend slowly roll out of the Shoulderstand, and relax completely.
10. Change places and reverse the posture.

"Put attention neither on pleasure or pain but 'between these.'"
Paul Reps, "Centering," ZEN FLESH, ZEN BONES

INVERTED POSTURES

Whenever we are tired we know how wonderful it feels to rest, to lie down, put our feet up, and close our eyes. We can actually feel the tiredness draining away as the blood flows out of our feet and circulates toward our head and heart.

Most of our life seems to be spent "on our feet." And if life is balance, then we need a daily period of being off of our feet.

To regain our lost vitality and to rejuvenate ourselves we need to experience the joys of Shoulderstand. The inverted position of the body in Shoulderstand reverses the internal organs. Taking the pressure off of the organs improves digestion, eases varicose veins and aids prolapsed organs.

The Shoulderstand increases the flow of blood to the brain which improves circulation to the throat and chest, relieves headaches, and soothes the nervous system. In the Shoulderstand the blood supply to the thyroid gland is increased. The thyroid gland which helps regulate body weight, growth, and metabolism is stimulated by tucking in the chin in the Shoulderstand. Stimulating and increasing the circulation to the thyroid gland helps to regulate and normalize it.

The benefits of Shoulderstand are increased when the pose can be held with ease and comfort. The warm, gentle but firm support of a friend makes the Shoulderstand a joyful as well as beneficial pose.

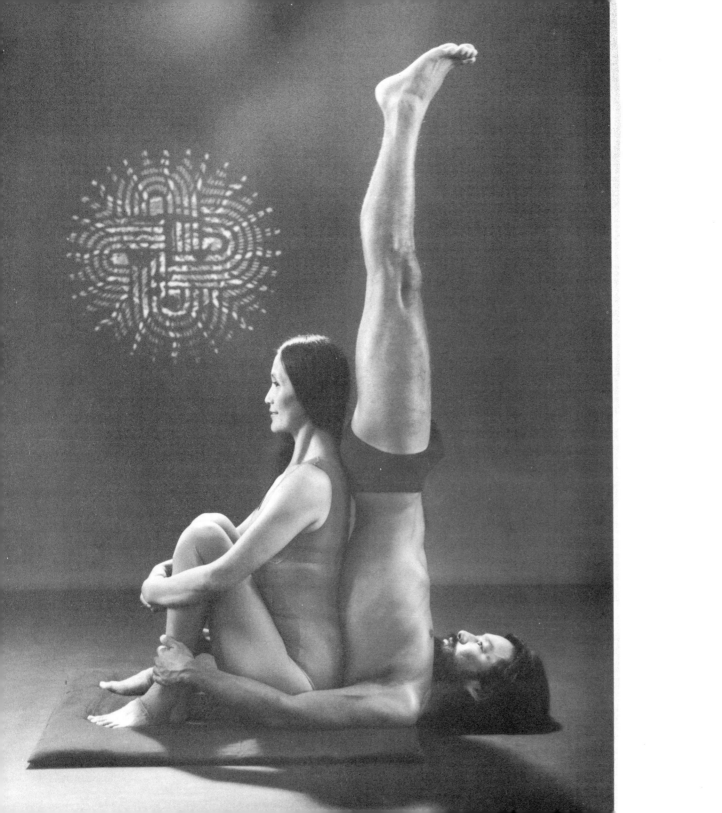

SHOULDERSTAND (Salamba Sarvangasana)

BEGINNING POSE: Recommended for all students with normal blood pressure.

BENEFITS: *The Shoulderstand improves circulation to the brain, relieves headaches, stimulates and normalizes the thyroid gland, aids digestion, and helps ease varicose veins.*

TECHNIQUE:

1. Lie flat on your back with your shoulders close to the edge of a folded blanket, hands at your sides, palms down.
2. Inhale, and while exhaling bend both knees, draw them toward your chest, and tuck in your chin.
3. With an exhalation press down with the palms, lift your hips, bring the knees toward the forehead, and support the back with your palms.
4. Inhale and lift the chest toward the chin. Exhale and straighten the legs. Breathe freely and naturally.
5. When you have reached your maximum lift, lower your arms to the mat with the hands shoulders-distance apart.
6. Allow your friend to sit as close to your back as possible with knees bent and feet flat. Hold your friend's ankles and rotate your shoulders under, stretching them away from your neck.
7. With arms circling knees, your partner lifts the chest, presses the base of the spine into your upper back, and moves the feet away keeping your arms taut.
8. Soften or close the eyes and experience together each other's warmth and support.
9. Release your friend's ankles, and as your partner moves aside, slowly roll down and rest.
10. Change places and reverse the pose.

"When there is complete understanding, there is silence."
O.M. Burke, AMONG THE DERVISHES

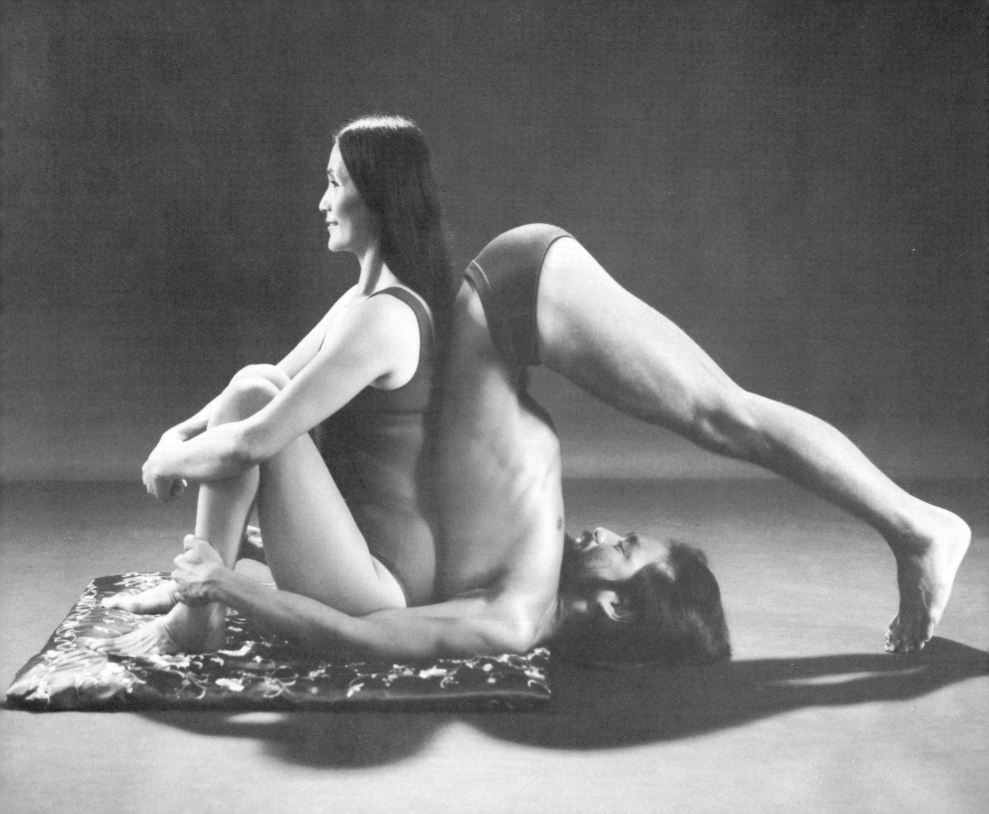

PLOUGH POSTURE (Halasana)

INTERMEDIATE POSE: Suitable for students with a limber spine and stretched-out leg muscles.

BENEFITS: *This pose stretches the hamstring muscles, massages the entire spine, eases backaches, and relieves stiffness in the shoulders.*

TECHNIQUE:
1. Lie flat on your back with your shoulders near the edge of a folded blanket, arms at your sides, palms flat, chin tucked in.
2. Inhale and press down with the palms. Exhale, bend the knees, lift the hips, and bring the knees toward the forehead. Rest the knees on the forehead for two breaths.
3. On an exhalation extend your legs and turn the toes under resting them on the rug.
4. Interlock the fingers behind your back, straighten your arms and squeeze your shoulder blades together as you expand your chest. Staying high on your toes, lift your hips and elongate your spine.
5. Release your hands and allow your partner to sit with knees bent and feet flat as close to your back as is possible.
6. Hold your partner's ankles and continue to rotate your shoulders under and stretch them away from your neck.
7. While your friend is pressing firmly into your upper back, lift your thighs, walk your feet nearer to your head, and come up onto the tips of your toes.
8. Hold, feeling your friend's back supporting your entire spine.
9. To release, let go of your partner's ankles, and as your friend moves aside, slowly roll down and relax.
10. Change places and reverse the posture.

"Awareness has no hands."
Tarthang Tulku, GESTURE OF BALANCE

INTEGRATION AND INVENTION IN YOGA

Accompanying the physical Yoga postures are two other elements of the science of Yoga which can be experienced together with a partner. They are breathing awareness and deep relaxation.

When the body, breath, and mind work together in a state of inner relaxation, a reintegration takes place which results in new growth for both partners.

At this point both friends are ready to experiment, to work together, and to develop new variations for the postures. Developing trust and cooperation allows the creative spirit within each of us to unfold.

BREATHING AWARENESS

Whenever we do Yoga postures with a friend correct breathing is included with each movement. Breathing awareness is central to the practice of Yoga. Yoga postures become more than mere exercises when we remain mindful of our breath. Coordinating movement with rhythmic breathing calms the mind and refreshes the spirit.

In this section two breathing practices are included which you and your partner may enjoy doing after you have completed the postures.

"Yogis count life not by number of years but number of breaths."
Swami Vishnudevananda, THE COMPLETE ILLUSTRATED BOOK OF YOGA

BASIC DEEP BREATHING – THE COMPLETE BREATH

BEGINNING POSE: Recommended for all students.

BENEFITS: Deep breathing nourishes and strengthens the respiratory system, removes toxins, clears and relaxes the mind, calms the emotions, and soothes the nerves.

TECHNIQUE:
1. Sit facing your friend a few feet apart on a rug and learn the practice of deep breathing together.
2. Fold your legs into a comfortable, cross-legged position. Rest your hands on your knees.
3. Inhale and straighten your spine; exhale and lower your shoulders keeping the spine erect. Soften the neck, relax the abdomen, and close the mouth. Exhale completely.
4. Beginning together, slowly inhale through the nostrils feeling the abdomen gently fill. As the breath rises allow your ribs to expand outward to the sides filling the lungs. Inhale completely and lift the chest while lowering and relaxing the shoulders.
5. Exhale completely through the nostrils as you contract your ribs slightly and pull in your abdomen.
6. Repeat the complete breath twice more with your partner.
7. Then relax together breathing freely and naturally.
8. Begin with three breaths daily. With consistent practice the number of complete breaths will gradually increase.

DEVELOPING MINDFULLNESS THROUGH BREATH AWARENESS

The concept of balance can be easily understood by observing the breathing process. The inhalations and exhalations are even and continuous. Whenever we are calm our breathing is slow and rhythmic. Exertion increases our rate of breathing and anxiety causes us to hold our breath. Remembering to breathe deeply in times of stress helps us to balance our emotions by balancing our breath.

The rhythmic movements of inhalation and exhalation have a calming effect on the mind. When we are conscious of our breathing our mind and body feel connected. Breathing awareness helps us to create a bridge from our outer body to our inner being.

"Whenever inbreath and outbreath fuse, at this instant touch the energyless energy-filled center."
Paul Reps, "Centering," ZEN FLESH, ZEN BONES

BREATH AWARENESS PRACTICE

BEGINNING PRACTICE: Recommended for all students.

BENEFITS: This practice develops attentiveness, concentration, and insight. It calms the mind, soothes the emotions, and turns the attention inward.

TECHNIQUE:
1. Sit several feet away from your friend on a rug.
2. Fold your legs into a comfortable, cross-legged position. Sit on a small pillow if you wish.
3. Rest the hands on the knees and close the eyes. Straighten the spine and lower the shoulders.
4. Breathe freely and naturally and begin to relax.
5. Keeping the eyes closed, sense the presence of your friend, and then turn your attention inward focusing on your breath.
6. At first be aware only of the rising and falling of the breath, the ''in and out'' movement of the abdomen.
7. As you become more and more alert follow the movements of your breath closely. Carefully notice the unique pattern of your breath, the pauses between breaths, and the many variations of the breath. Note that the breath can be rapid, calm, shallow, deep and that it is constant and yet changing.
8. Limit yourself to observing the breath and do not attempt to change it or to control it in any way.
9. When thoughts come into your mind, recognize them as thoughts, note them, and then return your attention to your breath. Do this gently over and over again, growing calmer, letting go of everything except the awareness of your breath.
10. After a few minutes slowly begin to return your attention to your surroundings and open your eyes. Quietly lie down and relax.

DEEP RELAXATION

Relaxation is a system of healing. Deep relaxation removes tiredness, eases anxiety, soothes nerves, and enables us to "let go."

The natural state of the body and mind is balance. Whenever we are truly relaxed we feel that inner balance. However, the world we live in produces tension in our lives. To relieve this tension we need to relearn proper relaxation.

Deep relaxation is not the same as sleep. Relaxation is a conscious process. Instead of entering the unconscious state of sleep, deep relaxation heightens our consciousness by expanding our inner feelings.

Relaxation needs to be practiced. Only when we have learned how to relax in a quiet room with our friend will we be ready to relax amid the tensions of the world. What is learned in stillness will be perfected in movement.

Deep relaxation naturally follows extension. It feels right to rest after doing Yoga poses together. Using the following deep relaxation procedure as a guide, enjoy relaxing with your friend.

"Everyone comes to Yoga to relax."
B.K.S. Iyengar, SPARKS OF DIVINITY

DEEP RELAXATION POSE (Savasana)

BEGINNING POSE: Recommended for all students.

BENEFITS: *This pose removes muscle fatigue, releases tension, soothes the nerves, and calms the mind.*

TECHNIQUE:

1. Lie flat on your back on a rug several feet away from your friend. With feet together, inhale and flex your feet; exhale and relax your hips as you separate your feet a few inches.

2. Rotate the shoulder blades under, rest your hands, palms up, a few inches from your sides. Align your head with your spine and close your eyes.

3. Begin to relax your body by directing your attention to your toes. Slowly allow your mind to travel up your body, part by part, noting any fatigue or tension. Direct your awareness to each part, letting go until the body has softened and the resistance has gone.

4. Center your attention on your breath. With each inhalation imagine your entire body filling with new energy. With each exhalation let go of anything you no longer need. Continue to inhale strength, peace, courage, and sufficiency and to exhale tiredness, tension, anger, and pain.

5. Now relax your breath and direct your mind to an image of the color red. Create an entire field of red. As soon as red becomes clear, slowly change the color to orange, to yellow, to green, to blue, and to violet. Experience each color fully noting the qualities these colors evoke within you. Finally allow violet to change into gold. Then observe the field of gold softening, melting. With your mind's eye imagine your entire body filling with liquid gold. At that moment feel the borders of your body slowly dissolve and the gold flow freely out into the universe.

6. Allow the peaceful feeling within you to expand. For a few moments live within that feeling of conscious relaxation.

7. After a few minutes gradually become aware of the sounds around you and your friend nearby. Slowly begin to enliven your body by deepening the breath, gently moving your toes, opening and closing your fingers, and rolling your head from side to side.

8. Roll onto your side and rest there, slowly opening your eyes. Take your time, there is no hurry. When you are ready, come to a sitting position. Pause for a moment allowing this feeling of relaxation to permeate your being.

INTEGRATION

"In order to develop higher awareness, we need to integrate the body, breath, and mind."

Tarthang Tulku, GESTURE OF BALANCE

When we study Yoga we begin with the body, for the body is what we know best. The postures teach us all we need to know about our physical being, our strengths and our weaknesses. Working with a friend helps us to open up our body, to free the tight places, to stretch further than ever before.

As we progress with the postures we add awareness of the breath. Correct breathing accompanies each pose. Breathing as we move improves the stretch, relieves the pain, and increases the expansion. However, the benefits of correct breathing are not only limited to the physical body. Breath is the integrating factor, the essence which coordinates the body with the mind.

Deep breathing relaxes our body and calms our mind. When we are truly relaxed, we experience a feeling of openness and a flow of inner energy.

The integration of the body and mind through the breath creates a state of inner balance. Within this moment of balance mind pressures cease and a feeling of satisfaction is experienced.

EXPERIMENTATION

"Yoga says to experience . . . Experiment and experience are both the same, only their directions are different. Experiment means something you do outwardly; experience means something you do inwardly. Experience is an inner experiment."

Bhagwan Shree Rajneesh, YOGA: THE ALPHA AND THE OMEGA

The reason Yoga works so well is that it is something you have to do. You don't become a balanced person by reading about Yoga or by believing in it; instead Yoga must be experienced.

Partnering in Yoga begins as an experiment. You and your friend may feel self-conscious at first. As you practice the postures together, learn deep breathing, and discover how to relax, your self-consciousness slowly dissolves.

While working together with your friend you will gradually realize that what you are creating with your bodies is balance. When you and your friend are open and receptive to each other, new variations will naturally emerge from the creative energy flowing between you.

What begins as a physical experiment becomes an inner experience.

GROWTH

"The goal of life is learning."
A. Sujata, BEGINNING TO SEE

Our experiences shape our perception, the way we view life. Each experience we share with a friend provides us with new insights, a glimpse of our own reality.

If we view life as offering us chances to grow, then our friends play a special part in this process.

A friend may be described as someone who is on your side, and whenever we work with someone who supports us, growth naturally occurs.

Yoga with a friend is a learning experience which teaches us to trust and rely on each other and helps us to nourish our inner growth.

SPECIAL REFERENCES

Burke, O.M. AMONG THE DERVISHES. New York: E.P. Dutton & Co., 1975.

Erhard, Werner. IF GOD HAD MEANT MAN TO FLY, HE WOULD HAVE GIVEN HIM WINGS. Werner Erhard, 1973.

Iyengar, B.K.S. BODY THE SHRINE, YOGA THY LIGHT. Bombay, India: Taraporewala, 1978.

Iyengar, B.K.S. LIGHT ON YOGA. New York: Schocken Books, 1966.

Luby, Sue. HATHA YOGA FOR TOTAL HEALTH. Englewood Cliffs, New Jersey: Prentice-Hall, Inc., 1977.

Rajneesh, Bhagwan Shree. YOGA: THE ALPHA AND THE OMEGA, Volume One. Poona, India: Rajneesh Foundation, 1976.

Reps, Paul, ed. "Centering," ZEN FLESH, ZEN BONES. New York: Anchor Books, Doubleday & Company, Inc.

Shain, Merle. WHEN LOVERS ARE FRIENDS. Philadelphia: J.B. Lippincott Company, 1978.

Smith, Adam. POWERS OF MIND. New York: Ballantine Books, Random House, Inc., 1975.

Stearn, Jess. YOGA, YOUTH, AND REINCARNATION. New York: Bantam Books, Doubleday & Company, Inc., 1965.

Sujata, A. BEGINNING TO SEE. Santa Cruz, California: Unity Press, 1975.

Tulku, Tarthang. GESTURE OF BALANCE. Emeryville, California: Dharma Publishing, 1977.

van de Wetering, Janwillem. A GLIMPSE OF NOTHINGNESS. Boston: Houghton Mifflin Company, 1975.

Vishnudevananda, Swami. THE COMPLETE ILLUSTRATED BOOK OF YOGA. New York: Pocket Books, Simon & Schuster, Inc., 1972.

Sandra Jordan currently teaches Hatha Yoga classes at the Silent Dance Center in Honolulu, Hawaii, a center for Hatha Yoga, Tai Chi Chuan, and other dance forms which she has managed since 1976. She received a B.A. degree in German and English from the University of California at Berkeley in 1962. After teaching elementary and junior high school in the Oakland and Berkeley areas, she spent 1966-1968 as a Peace Corps Volunteer in Barbados, West Indies. An avid world traveler and skilled photographer, she has exhibited her color and black and white photographs of Europe and India at the Kahala Mall in Honolulu. During 1977-1979 she undertook advanced study in the BKS Iyanger method of Hatha Yoga with Judith Lassiter and Ramanand Patel of California and Diana Clifton of England. She lives in Hawaii with her husband and two sons, and, in addition to teaching Hatha Yoga, freelances as a photographer and studies ballet.

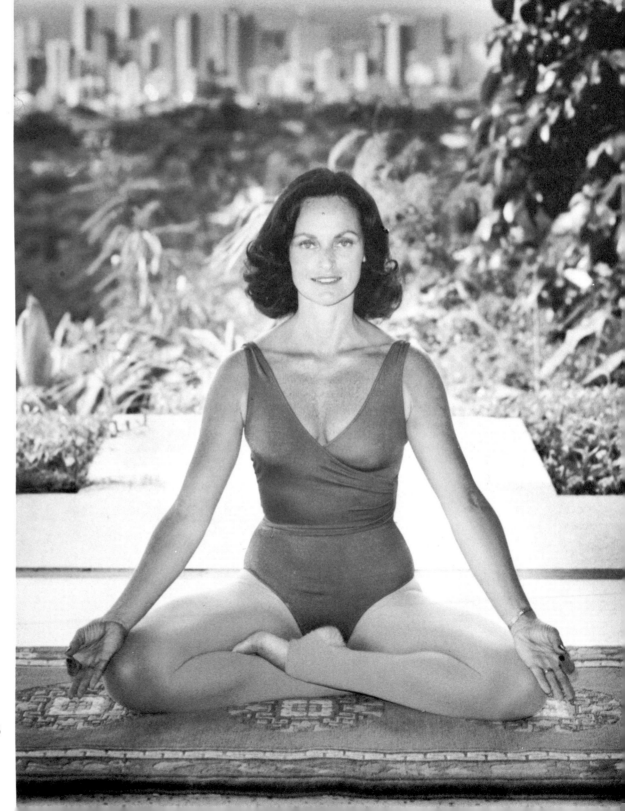